Self-discipline–the foundation for accomplishment and happiness.

Training means regularly practicing a course of action or a set of instructions in order to reach a desired goal. That's what discipline is all about. In the following pages, Dale Galloway assures you that by controlling yourself you're not missing out on anything, but getting ready for the very best. The theme "deny the lesser to gain the greater" is threaded throughout this book and applied to each subject covered. Dale Galloway's proven advice and practical directions will help you gain control of undisciplined areas of your life... acquire responsibility...have victory over temptation...and develop life-changing attitudes of success.

Dare to DISCIPLINE Yourself

Dale E. Galloway

Power Books

Fleming H. Revell Company
Old Tappan, New Jersey

Copyright © 1980, 1984 by Dale E. Galloway
Published by Fleming H. Revell Company
All rights reserved
Printed in the United States of America

Library of Congress Cataloging in Publication Data

Galloway, Dale E.
    Dare to discipline yourself.

    1. Christian life—1960–
BV4501.2.G287 1983   248.4   83-9716
ISBN 0-8007-5129-9

I dedicate this book to my beloved friends and staff pastors in the ministry of New Hope Community Church: Pastor Rich Kraljev and Pastor Jerry Schmidt.

Contents

Dare to Discipline Yourself

1

The Ingredient for Achievement

In 1956 I entered Olivet Nazarene College in Kankakee, Illinois, as a green freshman. The experience of living on the fourth floor of a freshman dormitory was an education in itself. A couple of doors from me lived a young man from the heart of the Midwest who from all appearances had it made. He came from an extremely wealthy family and while most of the rest of us worked our way through college, he played. There seemed to be no limit to the amount of spending money that he enjoyed.

My college schedule was that I would go to school from seven o'clock in the morning until about three o'clock in the afternoon. Then I would go to work and work until ten or eleven o'clock at night. Then I would study until I fell asleep. Almost every night without exception, about the time I would start studying, my rich friend down the hall would be leading the noise parade. His life was totally undisciplined. Not only did he not bother to study, he hardly ever went to class.

I'll never forget when the grades came out for the first semester. The boy with the golden opportunity to get a college education flunked out. All the time he should have been succeeding, he was failing. There was something awfully important missing in his life. This missing ingredient caused him to blow his educational opportunity.

Nancy Lambert has prided herself for years on being a night person. She brags to friends that she is wide-awake and going strong at the midnight hour. She even pokes fun at her husband, Ted, for going to bed early and leaving her up by herself. The catch is that she can never get herself out of bed in the morning. For years her three children and her husband have gotten their own breakfasts, such as they are, and gotten themselves off to work and school. Nancy has soothed her conscience by telling herself that her three children and husband don't need much of a breakfast anyway. And after all, they don't complain much anymore, so why should she struggle to be any different?

How shortsighted this mother has allowed herself to become. In giving in to her natural inclination to sleep in every morning, Nancy is missing the opportunity of preparing a nutritional breakfast for her family and sending them off to a good start. The bare truth is that these same children who are not supposed to care much always eat a hearty breakfast when someone is there to prepare it for them. Only Ted, Nancy's husband, can tell how many mornings he has trudged off to work with an unfulfilled need for companionship and communication with his wife. Because of a missing ingredient in Nancy's life, she is shortchanging her children, not meeting the need of her husband, and most of all settling for less than what is her best.

By discovering the missing ingredient and starting to use it in her life, Nancy could immediately begin succeeding where she is now failing. And so can you.

My friend, you do not have to blow your opportunities. You have within you what it takes if you will discover it and use it. This decisive ingredient for achievement does not have to be missing in your life. It can be yours. And when you discover it, cultivate it, and use it, it will serve you well by enriching your life with a trophy case full of personal achievements.

If you:

- are not getting what you want most
- feel like you are losing control over your own life
- find yourself surrendering the leadership of your life to runaway emotions and moods

THEN YOU NEED IT!

If you:

- have a desire for worthwhile achievement
- wish you could control your sex life
- want to get a handle on your anger
- need to master your moods
- long to succeed where you have been failing

THEN YOU NEED IT!

Without it:

- we eat too much and become fat
- we become morally weak and commit sex sins
- we become intellectually dull and stop expanding our horizons
- we become enslaved to habits that harm us
- we allow bad moods to master us and make us miserable companions
- we are overrun by negative emotions, which give rise to

destructive behavior and wreak havoc in our relationships with others
- we keep spending more money than we make and get
into financial messes
- we fail to achieve our dreams

What is it? What is this ingredient that is seriously lacking
in most people's lives today? There is no achievement without it. *What is it? It is self-discipline!*
Self-discipline can be the key that opens all doors to bring
you the things you truly want in life. With self-discipline
you can control your life rather than your life being out of
control. *You can take charge of your life and achieve.*
In this book I am going to open your eyes to the key of
self-discipline that you hold in your hands. Step-by-step, I
am going to show you how you can use self-discipline to
achieve those things that you've always wanted. Believe
me—personal achievement can be yours!

Something Everybody Needs and Nobody Wants

Self-discipline is what many of us need most and want
least. If we need it so much, then why do we resist it?
The first reason is because we all have a natural inclination to be lazy. There is within us a pull toward taking the
path of least resistance. If we did what we felt like doing, a
lot of the time we would end up doing nothing. So then if we
are to get the best things in life, we cannot give in to our own
laziness. As the greatest book of wisdom ever written, the
Bible, says: "Lazy people want much but get little, while the
diligent are prospering" (Proverbs 13:4 TLB). As someone
has said, "Temptation to laziness never grows old."

In order to get the best things out of life, in order to achieve the most worthwhile things, you must stand up to the lure of laziness. Take yourself in tow. Make yourself stand up and put one foot in front of the other. One thing is certain, if you don't take charge over your own life and manage it, no one will do it for you. A self-disciplined person is one who first conquers his own laziness.

The second reason that so many people resist self-discipline, I believe, is that they do not understand what self-discipline really is.

I can remember a time in my life when I didn't even like the word *discipline*. Something within me rebelled against it. When I was a student in seminary, I had a particular professor who would admonish us on the importance of self-discipline in our lives. Every time he would start into his little talk, my rebellion against the word *discipline* would turn him off. Then he wrote a book on the subject, and out of loyalty to him I read his book, but rebelled against every page I read.

Ten years later I picked up the same book and reread it. This time, to my utter amazement, I thought it was great stuff! What was the difference? The difference was that I had finally opened my mind to the areas of my life that were undisciplined. I also realized that if I was going to achieve the beautiful dreams that God had given to me, I needed to improve in the area of discipline.

Without Self-discipline There Can Be No Worthwhile Achievements

All the great achievers whom I have ever known personally have been men and women who have first learned to use discipline to master themselves. Self-mastery is the prerequisite for all worthwhile achievement. No one can expect to excel in his vocation until first he has gained control over himself. How can one even achieve in a marriage relationship until first he learns to control and master himself? Show me a marriage that's failing, and I'll show you one or two marriage partners whose lives are out of control. It is self-discipline that brings the best out of us.

The Bible says it this way: "To win the contest you must deny yourselves many things that would keep you from doing your best" (1 Corinthians 9:25 TLB).

The Apostle Paul further explains!

> To win the contest you must deny yourselves many things that would keep you from doing your best. An athlete goes to all this trouble just to win a blue ribbon or a silver cup, but we do it for a heavenly reward that never disappears. So I run straight to the goal with purpose in every step. I fight to win. I'm not just shadow-boxing or playing around. Like an athlete I punish my body, treating it roughly, training it to do what it should, not what it wants to. Otherwise, I fear that after enlisting others for the race, I myself might be declared unfit and ordered to stand aside.
>
> 1 Corinthians 9:25–27 TLB

From Paul's own personal experience and testimony comes this achiever's principle and theme of this very important book that we all need to make application of in our life. Here is the positive self-discipline princple: *Deny the lesser to gain the greater.*

Defining Self-discipline in a New, Positive Way

Contrary to what some people mistakenly think, *discipline* is not a negative word, but a positive one. It is best understood not as an end in itself but as a means to a desirable end. Self-discipline is a necessary exercise needed to fulfill a goal. Self-discipline is the way to improve yourself. It not only requires denying the lesser to gain the greater, but often means making the best choice between better and best. When self-discipline is at work, it chooses the best and ushers in a harvest of rich benefits. Self-discipline is the arrow that keeps us on target.

Recently when I looked up the synonyms for the word *discipline,* I discovered words like these: preparation, development, exercise, and training. Self-discipline is not:

- merely restraint, but preparation for release
- loss of freedom, but the road to greater freedom
- holding back, but moving ahead
- an enemy, but a friend
- self-punishment, but self-control
- slavery, but mastery
- an end in itself, but the beginning and follow-through to all worthwhile achievement

Positive Discipline for a Purpose

To get the best things in life there is a price to be paid. In the 1976 Olympic Games, held in Montreal, it was indeed a moment to cheer when twenty-six-year-old Bruce Jenner won the grueling ten-day decathlon competition and was acclaimed the world's greatest athlete.

This moment of personal victory and world triumph did not come easily. Jenner had trained long and hard for the decathlon after he finished ninth in 1972 in Munich. It was reported by sportswriters that he trained with nonstop dedication for more than seven hours a day for four years. Now that's self-discipline. Think of what this young man denied himself in order to become the world's greatest athlete. But in the moment of triumph all the hours of discipline were forgotten, and he only knew the glory of achievement. The Bible says it this way: "To win the contest you must deny yourselves many things that would keep you from doing your best" (1 Corinthians 9:25 TLB).

The chances are that you will not be a runner in the Olympic decathlon. But you, too, can be an achiever. The whole world of achievement belongs to the person who will put forth the willpower to discipline himself. It is that self-discipline that makes the mind sharp and quicker in its thinking processes. It is the self-disciplined body that has more energy and zest to keep going when others wear out. It is the one who has learned to control his emotions who keeps his cool when all others lose their heads. Self-discipline can shape you up until you feel like a champ instead of a chump.

Four Steps to Greater Achievements

1. WAKE UP TO YOUR NEED FOR SELF-DISCIPLINE. In the hotel there was a card to hang on the door whenever an individual wished to sleep late. In bold letters it said: PLEASE LET ME SLEEP. I can understand why someone might like to sleep

in once in a while, but to go through life asleep is a bad thing to do. Wake up! Wake up and admit to yourself the areas of your life in which you urgently need more self-discipline.

2. RECOGNIZE THERE ARE NO SHORTCUTS.   So often we human beings want achievement without first making the investment. We want the fruit of labors without putting in the labor. We want the butter without first churning the cream.

Great achievements come through self-discipline. Thomas Edison failed ten thousand times to create the light bulb. When asked how he felt about this, he said, "I didn't fail ten thousand times. I just found out ten thousand ways it wouldn't work!" You see, achievement comes through self-discipline. And let's face it, self-discipline is hard work. To become a self-disciplined person you have to put forth the effort not once, not twice, but again and again. *Deny the lesser to gain the greater.*

3. FIND MOTIVATION FOR SELF-DISCIPLINE FROM A PERSONAL ENCOUNTER WITH JESUS CHRIST.   As a young teenager I was an undisciplined person. My folks disciplined me, but there was little or no self-discipline inside me. I was drifting through life, often putting my worst foot forward, forfeiting the opportunities for learning that were mine, wasting my God-given potential.

Then I invited Jesus Christ to come into my life. I don't understand all that happened, but I know that when I went back to school in September, after having received Jesus two months before, my grades were immediately transformed from barely getting by to being an honor student. What made the difference? Jesus gave me the inner motivation to deny the lesser to gain the greater.

Our youth pastor, Dennis Hayes, is a young man who is studying to be a minister. Dennis has one of the finest personalities that I have ever run into in a young man. The people of the church really love him! Dennis comes from a family of five boys. The father and mother of these five have done a superb job of raising self-confident, motivated young men.

Dennis's father, Dan Hayes, was brought up as a migrant worker in California. Previous to his eighteenth birthday he didn't know what it was to go to sleep at night without the feeling of hunger in the pit of his stomach. He was brought up surrounded by illiteracy and poverty. Today he is a very cultured, educated, successful man who excels in his occupation and as a husband and father.

One day when Dan and I were having lunch together, I asked my friend, "How did you get out of that poverty rut to achieve the successful life that you now enjoy?"

He answered that at thirteen years of age he experienced the miracle of being born again. At his personal invitation, Jesus came into his life, accepted him just as he was, and said, "Let's go together from here to make something of your life." With the coming of the Lord Jesus into the center of his being came an inner dynamo of motivation to better himself.

You, too, can be motivated to better yourself by coming to know the more excellent one, Jesus, personally. Unfortunately, there are people who have become followers of Jesus who have yet to fully comprehend His call to a more excellent life. No Christian has to drudge along being unmotivated.

As we invite Jesus Christ to come into our life and fully cooperate with the good work He wants to complete within us (Philippians 1:6) it will give our life the lift upward. Fellowshiping with Jesus on a daily basis is the most inspiring and motivating experience that can happen in your life.

LOSE YOURSELF IN JESUS
and
YOU WILL FIND YOUR BETTER SELF.

4. BEGIN TO BECOME DISCIPLINED IN LITTLE, DAILY THINGS OF LIFE. Having determined to become a disciplined person, begin with the simple things. Start making your own bed promptly and neatly. Hang up your own clothes, clean up after yourself in the bathroom, start being on time for your appointments.

Beginning to become more disciplined in the small, daily things of your life will give you the willpower to become more disciplined in the areas that have been more difficult for you to master.

I love so much to eat that it makes it difficult for me to discipline my eating habits. But the interesting thing is, when I put forth the discipline to jog on a regular basis, I then find the willpower to discipline my eating habits. And the delightful result is physical fitness and a tight tummy instead of a flabby one.

Discipline can be likened to a muscle, in that the more you use it, the more strength you have to accomplish what it is you desire to do.

Self-discipline is a choice. After many conscious choices, it can become a beautiful habit. It can work for you without you even having to think about it. But let's face it, self-discipline will be a missing ingredient in your life unless you will it into action and persist in willing it into repeated action.

When I was a teenage boy, someone gave me a copy of the book *I Dare You!* by William H. Danforth. This challenging book begins with Mr. Danforth's own story:

As a small boy, before the time of drainage ditches, I lived in the country surrounded by swamp lands. Those were days of chills and fever and malaria. When I came to the city to school, I was sallow-cheeked and hollow-chested. One of my teachers, George Warren Krall, was what we then called a health crank. We laughed at his ideas. They went in one ear and came out the other. But George Warren Krall never let up. One day he seemed to single me out personally. With flashing eye and in tones that I will never forget, he looked straight at me and said, "I dare you to be the healthiest boy in the class."

That brought me up with a jar. Around me were boys all stronger and more robust than I. To be the healthiest boy in the class when I was thin and sallow and imagined at least that I was full of swamp poisons! The man was crazy. But I was brought up to take dares. His voice went on. He pointed directly at me, "I dare you to fill your body with fresh air, pure water, wholesome food, and daily exercise until your cheeks are rosy, your chest full, and your limbs sturdy."

As he talked, something seemed to happen inside me. My blood was up. It answered the dare and surged all through my body into tingling finger tips as though itching for battle.

I chased the poisons out of my system, I built a body that has equalled the strongest boys in that class, and has outlived and outlasted most of them. Since that day, I haven't lost any time on account of sickness. You can imagine how often I have blessed that teacher who dared a sallow-cheeked boy to be the healthiest in the class.

William Danforth was the founder of Ralston Purina and a vastly successful man. Not only was he a great success as an industrialist, but his inspiring book and talks motivated and inspired many people to become achievers. In the foreword to Mr. Danforth's book *I Dare You!* his friend, G. M. Philpott, writes:

Mr. Danforth always gave the best that was in him, whether he was guiding a great industry, travelling in a remote corner of the world, shooting ducks or playing with his grandchildren. The day ahead was always the most thrilling day in his life. The job at hand was always the most important one that he had ever undertaken. He never gave less than his best.

That is exactly what positive self-discipline is—giving whatever you're doing your best shot.

Do you want the best out of life? You want to reap the

rich benefits of success? Is there something that you want to achieve? Then I dare you to step out from the masses and:

DENY THE LESSER TO GAIN THE GREATER AND ENJOY BECOMING A SELF-DISCIPLINED ACHIEVER

Self-evaluation

1. Define *self-discipline* in your own words.

2. Take the self-discipline test by rating yourself on a scale from one to ten in the following areas (one being the lowest; ten being the highest).

   _____Exercise
   _____Sex life
   _____Habits that effect your health
   _____Choosing positive thoughts over negative ones
   _____Eating habits
   _____Moods
   _____Anger
   _____Finances
   _____Reading the Bible
   _____Emotional control
   _____Thought life

3. List the areas of your life in which you would like to become more disciplined.

4. What are the things that you would like to achieve that you could achieve through denying the lesser to gain the greater?

Six Steps to Get
What You Want Most

THE NEWSPAPER headlines made this astounding announcement, "Japanese Woman Scales Mt. Everest." For the first time in history a woman climber had conquered the world's highest mountain peak, which stands at 29,028 feet high. Mount Everest stands three times higher than Oregon's majestic Mount Hood. It is unbelievable but true: thirty-year-old Junko Tabei conquered the most unconquerable mountain in the world.

Before leaving on this historic climb, Mrs. Tabei had this to say to reporters, "Women are not so strong as men, but we can also climb the mountain slowly. Now I think only of climbing. Let us not talk of anything else."

How did Junko achieve what no other woman before her was ever able to achieve? Behind the scenes were years of preparation made up of training, discipline, and undying determination. No way could she have achieved this great accomplishment without years of self-discipline. Because she denied the lesser, she was able to climb the heights to gain this great accomplishment. Can you imagine the thrill and the sense of accomplishment Junko Tabei felt when she took that last step and climbed on top of the highest peak?

At that splendid moment it was worth everything it cost her
to make the trip to the top.

YOU, TOO, CAN CLIMB TO THE TOP.
YOU CAN CONQUER WHAT APPEARS TO BE AN
UNCONQUERABLE MOUNTAIN.
YOU CAN GET WHAT YOU WANT MOST—
IF YOU GO AFTER IT WITH EVERYTHING YOU'VE
GOT.

Today I stand in the middle of getting what I want most.
Approaching our eleventh anniversary celebration of New
Hope Community Church, it is thrilling to see what God has
done; out of nothing God has created something wonderful.
Eleven years ago, New Hope was only a dream that God
had planted in my heart and mind, which I shared with my
closest and best friend, my wife, Margi. At that time we had
no people, no money, no backing, but we had something
greater: a big vision of what God wanted to do through us to
take healing and hope to the unchurched thousands. Today
we minister to 3,000 to 4,000 people on an average Sunday.

On that first Sunday, October 14, 1972, when we drove together to the drive-in theater on Eighty-second Street in
Portland to launch a world ministry of inner healing and
hope, we were both excited and scared: excited about what
God, who can do the impossible, was going to do and
scared, in our humanness, that no one would show up and,
as some of our friends had predicted, we would fail. I
confess to you that it was a very humble beginning. But
at the same time, I was so consumed with the beautiful

dream I refused to look at the impossible odds against our success.

It was a moment I'll never forget when we leaned the ladder up against the roof of the snack shack. I pushed Margi first up the ladder, and then she pulled me up behind her. Sink or swim, we were partners in this exciting new ministry that God had given to us together. Little did we know how closely God would bind our lives together in love and ministry in the years to come.

As we walked across the roof of the snack shack, looked out to see our first fifty people, sang and preached, we began to put action into our dream.

In the first eight years of our ministry, we met in almost a dozen different facilities to conduct our New Hope Community Church services. When the winds of adversity came, as they did on many occasions, we were forced out, sold out, and on one occasion even burned out. Sometimes we were only given three days' notice to move. But each time we responded to adversity by looking for the striking opportunity and moved into a larger facility. And every place we moved not only did people follow us, but more people were added to the church daily.

Yes, there have been times when I have been tempted to give up. The going got tough. When the going gets tough, that's the time to get going. Every adversity we have used as a striking opportunity. Every setback, with God's help, we have turned into advance to do greater things for Him.

In February of 1981, we completed our first building, which seated 1,200 people. Located on thirteen prime acres on a hillside in the heart of Portland's freeway system, not only are we one block off the Sunnyside exit of Freeway 205 and on the high side of the freeway, but we are directly across from the largest shopping center in Oregon. No church ever had a more visible location that is accessible to hundreds of thousands of people. Already we are into four services on Sunday in order to handle thousands of people who are coming. We have just begun to realize our God-given dream. Our goal is to have 10,000 members by 1990; we have conceived, we believe it, and with God's help we are going to achieve it.

I believe that you, too, can see your dreams come true. You can set worthwhile goals and then see them accomplished with the discipline of using these six steps.

Step 1: Dare to Believe that You Can Achieve

How important is it to believe? Did you know that one entire gospel in the New Testament was written by John, the beloved disciple, in order that you might believe? The key verse of John's gospel says, "But these are written, that ye might believe that Jesus is the Christ, the Son of God; and that believing ye might have life through His name" (John 20:31 KJV). So significant is the word *believe* that it is used no less than ninety-eight times in John's gospel.

BELIEVE—*THE MAGIC WORD
THAT TRANSFORMS THE IMPOSSIBLE INTO THE
POSSIBLE.*

A few years ago I had the privilege of becoming personally acquainted with Lee Braxton. Lee is an inspiration to everyone who knows him as well as to anyone who has heard his story. Lee Braxton, of Whiteville, North Carolina, was the son of a struggling blacksmith. He was the tenth child in a family of twelve. ". . . so you might say," says Mr. Braxton, "that I became acquainted with poverty early in life. By hard work I managed to get through the sixth grade in school. I shined shoes, delivered groceries, sold newspapers, worked in a hosiery mill, washed automobiles, and served as a mechanic's helper."

Shortly after becoming a mechanic, Lee married. With his meager pay the family was having a tough time getting by. To add to their difficulties, Lee lost his job. Because he was unable to make the mortgage payment, his home was about to be taken away. It seemed like a hopeless poverty situation.

But if you know Lee Braxton, you know he's a man of character. He has a strong faith in Jesus Christ as his Lord. The more difficult things became, the more his belief level grew. Along with reading the Bible, he read books like *Think and Grow Rich*, which raised his belief level to an all-time high.

Lee dreamed his dream, set his goals and with tireless self-discipline, pursued the achieving of his objective. Lee Braxton organized the First National Bank of Whitefield and became its first president. Later he was elected mayor of the city. Lee aimed high—in fact, for the peak. He set as his goal to be rich enough to retire by age fifty. He achieved his goal six years ahead of time.

Since the age of forty-four he has been financially free to donate all of his skills, abilities and time to help make the ministry of Oral Roberts the tremendous success that it is today.

If you were to talk to Lee Braxton today, he would tell you that believing and acting on that belief is what made all the difference in his life.

Nothing worthwhile is ever accomplished until someone believes it can be done. It is absolutely amazing the mighty things God wants to do through our lives if only you will believe. Not just half-way believe, but *really* believe.

Someone said, "If you believe you can do something, you will never give up because of obstacles. If you believe you cannot do something, you will be more inclined to give up early."

How true! Without belief, not only do you give up early but often you don't even get off the starting block. *Believing is knowing that it can be done somehow, somewhere, and sometime.*

How pathetic to get caught in the "I can't do" trap. At times, we all fall into the "I can't" trap. "I can't do it"; "it can't be done." How many times have you said that to yourself or other people?

A middle-aged man, working long hours as a night watchman, on meager pay, told me that as a young man he had passed up a tremendous opportunity to learn and take over a thriving business. He explained that the reason he didn't go and seize the opportunity was that he lacked the belief in himself that he could do it. Now his past memories were filled with deep regrets. Whatever you do, don't let these sad words become your testimony: "It might have been."

I want you to ask yourself some very important questions. First question: *Am I willing to drift through life like the masses, putting forth little effort and accomplishing less?* If the

answer to this question is yes, then you have a problem. In
fact, in my opinion, to waste your life away like this is a sin.
The Bible says: "Therefore to him that knoweth to do good,
and doeth it not, to him it is sin" (James 4:17 KJV). You do
want to put forth the effort to get the best things in life, don't
you? If you do, then keep reading.

JESUS CAME TO PUT THE "CAN-DO" IN YOU. This is the
verse that He wants to put right inside the core of your
being, "I can do all things through Christ which strengtheneth me" (Philippians 4:13 KJV). I want you to ask yourself
this question: *With God as my help, what can I do?* The right
answer is found in Scripture: "With men this is impossible;
but with God all things are possible" (Matthew 19:26 KJV).
Say it: "With God's help, I can do it."

HOW CAN I DO THIS? Clifford Frazee was a very successful
businessman. In order for Cliff to make a success of his business, he often had to travel out of town for weeks at a time.
He loved his wife and four children so much that he just
hated to leave them for this period of time. But in order to
show his love to them, when he returned, he would always
bring gifts for the wife and each of the children.

The baby in the family was a seven-year-old girl who had
been involved in an accident and was confined to a wheelchair. Everyone in the family loved her in a special way, and
she was very close to her daddy. Every time her daddy came
home from work, he would pick her up and carry her
around the house on his back, and they would laugh and
enjoy the fun together. When her daddy had to be out of
town, he missed her, and she missed him very much.

This time he had been gone for two weeks and brought
home with him gifts for everyone as usual. But for his little

girl in the wheelchair he brought home a very special gift—a huge stuffed panda bear. The bear was as big as she was. As he handed it to his little girl, skeptically his wife said, "It's so big, how will she ever carry it?" As quick as a flash the happy little girl answered, "Mother, mother, I'll tell you how. I'll carry the bear, and daddy will carry me."

When you look at it from the human standpoint, it looks impossible. If you think it's impossible then you need to hear this power-packed verse. "I can do all things through Christ which strengtheneth me" (Philippians 4:13 KJV). I understand that you can't do it by yourself—but with Christ's help, it can be done. Jesus Christ has the ability to turn ordinary people into extraordinary human beings. As we allow Him to become Lord of our lives, He delights in releasing the best within us and adding His power to it; you doing your best plus God's power flowing through your life equals success.

WITH GOD'S HELP—YOU CAN DO IT!

In the early days of this ministry, after reading several inspirational self-help books, I was meditating on Philippians 4:13, when the Lord crystallized in my mind what I have since coined as our Achiever's Creed. Join the achievers by making this creed your motto:

WHATEVER THE MIND CAN CONCEIVE
AND I WILL DARE TO BELIEVE,
WITH GOD'S HELP, I CAN ACHIEVE.

Step 2: Dream a Lofty Dream

The Bible says, "Where there is no vision, the people perish" (Proverbs 29:18 KJV). Everyone needs a dream. Without a dream a person is not fully turned on to living. It is an all-inspiring dream that makes you bounce out of bed in the morning, heightens all your senses, and makes the creative juices flow. It is far better, I think, to live life to age thirty-five with a dream than to live life without a dream to age ninety-five.

Dreams lift us, inspire us, and put zest into our daily living. Wherever you are, whoever you are, whatever's happened in your life, whatever your age is now, it is not too late for you to dream a lofty dream. Catch hold of a dream and it will lift you to higher heights.

I believe that dreams are God-given gifts. Into every mind God drops beautiful ideas that, when received and nurtured, can bloom into beautiful dreams. To receive the dream you must take the blinders off and open up your mind to receive ideas.

TAKE THE LID OFF YOUR MIND. Have you heard about the jumping fleas? There were at least 10,000 fleas spread like a blanket across the teacher's desk. To entertain themselves they started playing a rather wild game called the jumping game. Higher and higher they jumped, again and again, trying to out jump the others. Up and down, up and down.

Then, the teacher sneaked up on them and covered them with a jar. Not knowing what had happened, they kept hitting their heads on the ceiling of the jar as they jumped up and down. But after being battered on the head a few times, they got the message and stopped jumping so high. They would still jump, but stop an inch from the top in their jump. After an hour the teacher removed the jar, but those fleas never knew the difference, because now in their minds they had fixed an imaginary ceiling. Although the jar was removed, they refused to try to jump any higher than the self-imposed barriers in their minds. How often we limit ourselves by the imaginary ceilings that we set in our minds.

Back as early as 1864 men were beginning to dream of running the four-minute mile. No one really believed it could be done, so for the next ninety years it didn't happen. But in the year 1954 a medical doctor expanded his mind and believed that he could run a four-minute mile; believing it, he did it. Once the barrier had been broken, do you know how many people ran a four-minute mile in the next two years? Now it took 100 years for one person to break the barrier, but believe it or not, in the next two years 163 people ran the mile in less than four minutes. What had happened? The limitation placed on the mind had been lifted. The most amazing things happen when we take the lid off our minds.

ASK YOURSELF THIS QUESTION: *With one life to live, what beautiful dreams do I want to fulfill in my lifetime?* If you could accomplish anything in this world that you wanted to accomplish, what would it be? One thing about it, it doesn't cost anything to dream, and it sure is a lot of fun. Besides, dreaming is the beginning of all worthwhile achieving. As Andrew Carnegie has said, "All achievement, all earned riches, had their beginning in an idea!"

Step 3: Decide What It Is You Want

Having opened your mind to consider infinite possibilities, things you want to achieve in your lifetime, ask yourself this question: *What are the things I really want most?* While you are thinking about it, get a sheet of paper and write those things down.

Right now I am thinking of the scores of people who drift through life aimlessly. Aiming at nothing worthwhile, they end up with what they aimed at—nothing worthwhile. Sure, they're dissatisfied with their meager results. Yet nothing is going to change until they decide to change it. Decide now that you are not going to be an aimless drifter but that you are going to use your God-given power of choice to decide what it is you want most and go after it.

To get the best results in your life I urge you to select only the most worthwhile dream. Unfortunately, there are some people who spend their lives dreaming dreams that aren't worth their time. I remember well a young man whom I counseled with a few years ago who spent a lot of time dreaming how he was going to win his best friend's wife and make her his wife. Needless to say, his dream turned into a nightmare. His dream, although somewhat exciting for him at the time, did not have any lasting value.

Test what it is you want by giving it the worthwhile test. Whenever I get a dream-inspiring idea that comes into my mind, I always ask myself these four questions:

1. Would this be a great thing for God?
2. Would it help hurting people? In other words, would it meet a human need?

3. Is it an idea that is inspiring?
4. Would it bring out the best in me?

If the answer is yes to all four questions, then you have the makings of a worthwhile achievement.

Why not go after the best things in life? Don't sell yourself short. To get the best, it is important that you see clearly what are the best things to go after in life. Doris Beasley not only made it a hobby to rummage through second-hand stores but had become something of an expert in spotting valuable antiques. In fact she got so good at it that she would discover valuable antiques being sold as junk. One Saturday as she was rummaging through a neighborhood run-down second-hand shop, she uncovered a valuable antique vase. It was so covered with dust and dirt, it appeared to be almost worthless. But, in the hands of the discerning antique buyer, as the dirt was rubbed away its true value was quickly spotted.

Doris made the purchase for $.25, took her valuable vase home, cleaned it up, and in a few days resold it for $500.00. How's that for a profit? Interestingly hundreds of people had gone through that same secondhand store, many of whom had even picked up the $.25 vase, yet because they didn't look beyond the surface, its true value remained hidden.

In our society today there are a lot of people who are settling for the lesser things of life. Drifting along in the masses, they are missing the things that are of the most value—many times right under their noses. Those things which are of the greatest value are to be found in knowing Jesus Christ and in understanding the Bible. It is these things that are eternal and will last when everything else has passed away. Jesus said it this way:

> Lay not up for yourself treasures upon earth, where moth and rust doth corrupt, and where thieves break through and steal: But lay up for yourselves treasures in heaven, where neither moth nor rust doth corrupt, and where thieves do not break through nor steal: For where your treasure is, there will your heart be also.
>
> Matthew 6:19–21 KJV

Have you heard about the world's greatest success principle? Here is the key to true, lasting success. "In everything you do, put God first, and he will direct you and crown your efforts with success" (Proverbs 3:6 TLB).

True success comes from putting God first, then establishing your priorities upon the foundation of our Lord's teachings in the Bible.

In the university of hard knocks, living in fellowship with Jesus as my Lord, and from application of the Bible have come a priority system of what matters most in my life. I share them with you that you might be challenged to establish your priority system built on the solid rock of Jesus as Lord and the Bible. Here they are:

First priority—My relationship with Jesus means more to me than anything else in my life.

Second priority—My love relationship with my wife and four children is more important to me than any other human relationship in life.

Third priority—The ministry of New Hope that God has given me to heal hurts and build dreams is something to

which I dedicate everything I have in order to excel in it.
Fourth priority—Friendships and relationships mean more to me than material things.
Fifth priority—Money is important to me for the good I can do with it. It is a gift from God to use and to give.

What matters most in your life? Do you have your priorities straight? With your priorities straight, you are now ready to crystallize into the form of a goal that which you want most in your life. Crystallize your goal.

Let me further illustrate the importance of each of us setting goals by sharing with you this story about a high school basketball team. Steve's burning ambition was to coach his high school basketball team to a state basketball championship. His dream became the dream of each of his players. The boys gave up their summer to play basketball for endless hours each day. As fall came, they gave up going out for the football team, so that they might further improve their basketball before the season opened. These boys even gave up going out with girls, so that they might think only of their single purpose of winning the state championship.

Basketball season opened with the team winning, and each game was one more victory in their march towards the crown. Now it is the night of the big game—the deciding game. If they win this one, they will be state champions. The teams finish their warm-up shots. They are physically ready for the game.

The team goes down to the locker room for one last pep talk from the coach. They don't really need the pep talk—the adrenaline is already flowing. It is obvious that the players are really up for this one. After the final shot in the arm, before the action begins, they charge out of the locker room—almost tearing the door off its hinges as they run onto the court. Abruptly, they stop in their tracks in complete confusion, which soon gives way to frustration and anger. They point out that the goals have been removed. They angrily demand to know how they can play a game without the goals. Everyone knows that you cannot play a basketball game without goals. I mean, how would you know the score? You wouldn't know if you hit the basket or not. You would have no way of knowing how you were doing. You see, if you're going to play a basketball game, you have to have goals to aim for.

How about you? Are you trying to play the game of life without goals? If you are, it is no wonder that you are frustrated. Is it surprising that you are failing to achieve?

NO GOALS—NO ACHIEVEMENTS!

The other day I was having lunch and fellowship with a fellow pastor in our city. As we were sharing together our various dreams and ministry, my new friend asked me this question. "Dale, if you were going to start New Hope Community Church again, what would you do differently from what you have done in the last eleven years?" I thought and thought. Do you know I couldn't come up with anything I would do differently. To tell you the truth, I felt that maybe I wasn't being humble to tell that to my friend. But I explained that the reason I wouldn't change anything is that the dreams and concepts were goals that I crystallized before the ministry ever started eleven years ago. For example, I visualized having 1,000 members in the first ten years. Not only do we have 1,000 members, but we had 550 additional ones, which gave us a total of 1,550 members in our first ten years.

You too can see great dreams come true, if you will take the time to not only visualize but crystallize your goals.

Step 4: Dive in and Get Started

I hate to admit how close I came to never launching the ministry of New Hope Community Church. You ask, "Didn't God give you a beautiful dream?" Yes, He did. "Then why did you almost not do it?" Because I was afraid of failure. In the midst of trying to decide whether to move ahead with my dream or run from the dream, I had the privilege of meeting with my friend Dr. Robert Schuller, who was visiting in our city of Portland. I asked the leading possibility thinker, himself, what I should do. Through no fault of Dr. Schuller's I left that day somewhat disappointed. Later I realized that what I wanted was someone who would guarantee me that if I pursued the dream, I would be successful. That was something no one could guarantee me.

Fortunately for me, a few days later, I was reading once again one of Dr. Schuller's books and I came across this famous line, which has come to mean so much to me in my pioneering of new ministries. Here it is:

I WOULD RATHER ATTEMPT TO DO SOMETHING GREAT FOR GOD AND FAIL THAN TO DO NOTHING AND SUCCEED

As I read these words they gripped my heart, and I made up my mind that the prize, if won, was well worth taking the risk. So that day I made up my mind that, sink or swim, I was going to go ahead and jump in. I set the date, October 14, 1972, to launch the ministry of New Hope Community Church. Nothing happened until I first set the date. After I set the date, all of my creative energies began to flow toward making the dream a reality. Someone has said that getting started is half the job.

During these eleven years of ministry of New Hope, we have never yet stopped risking failure. Every time we advance to move ahead to a new level of ministry, just like the turtle, we have to stick our necks out. But how full of adventure life is. I know that if we ever stop putting our necks out, it will be that day that we stop moving ahead to fulfill the big dreams that God gives to us to accomplish.

You want to fulfill a beautiful dream? Wipe out your fears with a strong faith in God and move ahead and get started now!

The story is told about a golfer who is repeatedly missing with a five-iron and hitting the ant hill. With every miss of the ball he slays another million or so ants. Getting a little frightened, one ant says to the other one, "We'd better get on the ball if we want to stay alive." The way to be filled with life is to get on the ball by getting started in going after what you want most.

I DARE YOU TO GET STARTED!

Step 5: Dedicate Yourself to Accomplish the Project

Dedicate yourself to fulfilling your dream. There is a price to be paid to fulfill a large dream. The bigger the dream, the bigger the price one must pay to see its fulfillment. One day a young man came to Jesus, wanting to have eternal life—a wonderful dream. Jesus plainly told him the price he would have to pay to have the fulfillment of eternal life. The young man, unwilling to pay the price, went away sorrowful and ended up the loser. A lot of people never achieve their dreams simply because they never dedicate themselves to put in the all-out effort to make their dreams a reality.

THERE IS NO FEAST WITHOUT A SACRIFICE.

No one has yet to ever get what they want most by wishful thinking. The best things come only to those who put forth the discipline of hard work. Some people foolishly kid themselves into believing that God is going to do for them something they can do for themselves. God, our Heavenly Father, will never do for us what we are able to do for ourselves. He is too wise for that. He knows that we need the discipline of doing our best to achieve not only the prize we're after but our own character building. Split the word *triumph* and you have tri-umph. It takes a whole lot of trying and an extra lot of umph to make dreams come true.

I have been very inspired by Rocky Bleier's story, so graphically written by Frank Gifford in *Gifford on Courage*. The story begins on January 7, 1968, with the teams of the National Football League holding their annual drafts of new players. Rocky Bleier, although a player from the famous school of Notre Dame, was not at the head of anyone's list. The truth was, he wasn't even on most of the team's wanted lists. As one scout said about him, "I don't think this boy can make a pro club." By some miracle he did get picked by the Pittsburgh Steelers. The Steelers picked eighteen players that year, and Rocky was number eighteen.

Before Rocky could get a chance to try out for professional career in football, he was drafted into the army and sent to Vietnam. Nine months later when he returned to the States, his right foot was half a shoe size smaller than his left; a grenade had exploded at his feet. The army listed Rocky Bleier as being 40% disabled. With the damage that had been done to the ligaments, tendons, and muscles in the foot, experts said that he would do well if he would ever be able to walk normally again.

As the wounds healed, Rocky began to work out by himself. The first time he tried to run, the pain was so excruciating that he collapsed. At this time Rocky could not walk or begin to run without suffering unbearable pain.

But this young man who had dedicated himself to the goal of becoming a professional football player refused to give up. He literally pulled himself out of bed at 5:00 A.M. and put will over pain as he ran for hours, up and down the steps of the Kansas State University football stadium. After running until he couldn't go any farther, he would go to the weight room for a grueling workout to build up his muscles.

Those first two years, when Rocky reported to football training camp, he just didn't have the physical capabilities to make the team. The coaches, the trainer and everyone else believed that Rocky's chance of ever playing professional football was zero. But Rocky set his jaw; he was determined that he was going to fulfill his dream of playing professional football.

During the off-season he took an apartment in Chicago. There in the chilly, windy city he would get up before dawn and run, run and run some more. With his determined mind he disciplined his body way beyond where it wanted to go. But as he kept pushing himself further and further, amazing things started happening. His body started responding by gaining strength. In the afternoons, Rocky worked selling insurance to pay the bills. At night, he would be back to the physical workout, doing three or four more hours of hard physical body building before collapsing into bed for another night's sleep.

After a couple years of this kind of rugged physical discipline, Rocky Bleier reported to football training camp. To everyone's amazement, the kid who never was supposed to be able to play professional football made the team. Unbelievable but true, his time in the forty-yard dash was clocked as faster than he was able to run before having part of his foot blown off by a grenade in Vietnam. Three years of committed, determined discipline were beginning to pay off for the tough kid who refused to give up this dream to play professional football. Rocky Bleier, the man they thought they were being kind to when they told him to quit, refused to give up his dream. From 1975–1980 Rocky Bleier blocked, ran the ball, and was one of the key persons in leading the Pittsburgh Steelers to the conquest of their dynasty of world championships. I salute Rocky Bleier, Superbowl champion, for his self-discipline.

Those who get the best things in life are those who are

dedicated to pay the price for success. You, too, can get what you want most if you will deny the lesser to gain the greater.

Step 6: Determine to Stick With It Until You Achieve It

One of the primary reasons so many people never achieve their dreams is that as soon as they suffer a little temporary setback, they give up.

It's been my observation that the achievers are just ordinary people who have made up their minds that what they are doing is worthwhile, and they stubbornly refuse to give up until they achieve their goal. Extraordinary projects are accomplished by ordinary people who refuse to give up.

Lee Braxton likes to tell this little story: A father was trying to encourage his discouraged son by saying:, "Don't give up—don't ever give up." The boy replied, "But I can't solve these math problems." The father replied, "Remember, son, the people who are remembered are those who didn't give up . . . Robert Fulton didn't give up, Thomas Edison never gave up, Eli Whitney never gave up, and look at Isadore McPringle." The boy said, "Who is Isadore McPringle?" "See," said the father, "you never heard of him. . . . He gave up."

If you are going to enjoy the riches of achieving worthwhile things in your life, you are going to have to overcome a lot of big obstacles. The more worthwhile thing you are trying to achieve, the bigger the obstacles. You can expect many difficulties along the road to your achievement. When the going gets tough, that's no time to panic, give up, throw in the towel. That's the time to toughen up. *When the going gets tough, with Christ's help, the tough get going!*

Sometimes achieving is slow going. It is in times like that when we are tempted to become discouraged and give up. Did you know the average speed of the Santa Maria during the voyage across the Atlantic was just two miles an hour? That was slow enough to discourage even the hardiest and most seasoned sailor. Added to the snail's pace were all the forceful winds and rolling sea. Yet through it all Columbus kept the ship moving in the direction of his dream. Courageously, Columbus and the crew persisted against the most adverse conditions. They pressed on. Refusing to give up, they discovered America.

"BRAVE ADM'R'L, SAY BUT ONE GOOD WORD:
WHAT SHALL WE DO WHEN HOPE IS GONE?"
THE WORDS LEAP LIKE A LEAPING SWORD:
"SAIL ON! SAIL ON! SAIL ON! AND ON!"

JOAQUIN MILLER
"Columbus"

Today are you in a tough spot? Things look impossible? You feel like quitting and giving up? Do you remember what General Douglas MacArthur said when his forces in Korea were suffering setbacks until they were backed up against the sea? Someone asked the general what he thought of the desperate situation, and he replied with strong words. "I have never been more confident of victory than I am today." He was right. Before long, the tide turned. He led his forces through it all to victory.

There is a great General who can help you. He's not just any old five-star general, He is the Chief and Commander of

Forces of God. His name is *Jesus.* He is our Leader. Look to Jesus! Follow Him! He will bring you through to victory!

"I can do all things through Christ which strengtheneth me."

> WITH GOD'S HELP
>   YOU CAN CONCEIVE,
>   YOU CAN DARE TO BELIEVE,
>   AND YOU CAN ACHIEVE.

Three Principles for Better Health and More Energy

"WHAT IS good health?" I asked a mother of three small children the other day. She said, "To me, good health is being able to get out of bed in the morning and make it through another day." I asked a middle-aged executive what he thought was good health, and he said, "I haven't been to the doctor in three years, so I consider myself in good health."

What do you think of when you think of the words *good health?* Is good health not being sick or maybe only having one headache a week? Does the mere absence of sickness mean a person is in good health? If you think good health is only the absence of sickness, then you are cheating yourself by clinging to a very small concept of good health.

Good health is so much more than the mere absence of disease and sickness. It includes full, deep breaths, a spring in your step, energy to tackle big problems, strength to keep going with zest when other people are tired and worn out.

God's wish is for your good health and high energy level: "Beloved, I wish above all things that thou mayest prosper and be in health, even as thy soul prospereth" (3 John 2 KJV).

The Old Testament is full of detailed provisions and rules for good health. A large portion of the Book of Leviticus is devoted to the health and welfare of God's people. For example, guidance was given as to what meats to eat and what meats were unclean (Leviticus 11). We now understand from modern science that the meats designated as unclean were probably highly contaminated.

In Numbers 19 and Deuteronomy 23, the children of Israel are told how to purify themselves after touching a dead body. They are given explicit instructions on repeated washings with running water, with time spent in between drying their hands in the sun to kill bacteria. God gave them the law, and when they obeyed it, they were protected from the germs that spread diseases, although they didn't know anything about bacteria.

Long before modern science discovered the importance of sanitation for good health, God told His people what to do: "You shall set off a place outside the camp and, when you go out to use it, you must carry a spade among your gear and dig a hole, have easement, and turn to cover the excrement" (Deuteronomy 23:12, 13 BERKELEY).

Throughout the Bible it is proven again and again how concerned God is for our physical health and well-being as a people. All of His Commandments given to us to obey are for our own well-being and good physical, mental, and emotional health.

Contrary to what some people might think, God is not one who will do everything for us. He will not do for us what we can do for ourself. To each of us, God has given responsibility of caring for the health and welfare of our own bodies and minds. Someone has said, "Your life is a gift from God; what you do with your life is your gift back to God."

In other words, God has given to you the responsibility of taking care of yourself. If you do a good job, you will reap rich rewards of good health and abounding energy, beginning here and now. If you don't take yourself in hand and practice self-discipline, then you will drag through life wishing you felt better.

I can remember how excited I was to be a member of the Mifflin High School football team. To be on the team and play football had been a dream of mine from a very early age. When I made the team, I had such a desire to play that I was willing to do whatever the coach told me. If he suggested that we eat particular foods, that's what I ate. When he told us to go to bed early, that's what I did. In the springtime, when he would lay out an exercise program for us for the summer so we would report to training camp in good shape, I followed it to the letter. I was willing to pay any price because I wanted the experience of being on a winning football team.

High school days have come and gone a long time ago. In these years that have followed I have discovered there is a far bigger game than football. It is the game of life. I've also discovered that to succeed in the game of life it is just as essential to be physically fit as it was to succeed in the game of football. If one pays the price of self-discipline to make his mind and body fit, he will reap the rich rewards of good health and high energy output. On the other hand, if any one of us allows himself to drift along in an undisciplined flabby existence, he will reap the consequences of bad health that become like a lead pipe hanging around his neck.

Now I am going to share with you three principles to help you to not only keep free from diseases of the mind and body but to release the flow of boundless energies. To treat yourself to good health and more energy, practice these three positive principles:

Principle 1: Take Charge of What You Eat

Your body is the temple of God.

Haven't you yet learned that your body is the home of the Holy Spirit God gave you, and that he lives within you? Your own body does not belong to you. For God has bought you with a great price. So use every part of your body to give glory back to God, because he owns it."

1 Corinthians 6:19, 20 TLB

How well are you taking care of the temple of God—your body? Is it in tip-top condition, or is it run down? It is tragic to see so many people abusing the temple of God.

To start with, I want to ask you a penetrating question that at first may seem almost humorous. Here it is: *Why do you eat?* After asking myself this same question recently, I discovered I eat to satisfy my hunger. I eat out of habit. I eat to please my taste buds. All too often appetite has governed what I have eaten and how much.

I've come to a brand-new realization concerning eating: Good health, not appetite, should be the number one purpose for our eating.

"Animals feed, man eats; the man of intellect alone knows how to eat" (Anthelme Brillat-Savarin). Begin gaining mastery over life by first mastering what you eat. Your diet governs how you act, look, and feel. As Howard Long, president of American Physical Fitness Institute of Los Angeles, said, "Sound nutrition does have a dynamic and lasting effect on health."

Proper nutrition, which can be had only through a balanced diet, can:

- Contribute to your mental stability
- Greatly reduce heart problems
- Keep your arteries cleaned out and functioning
- Defend against diseases
- Hasten convalescence
- Give you a strong body
- Add luster, vitality, and energy to your daily life

To feel right, you must first eat right. Back in Old Testament times, God told the children of Israel not to eat fat from animals (*see* Leviticus 3:17; 7:23, 24). This was thousands of years before modern science told us about the cholesterol problem in the blood that can come as a result of eating too much animal fat. Nutritionists tell us that nine out of ten Americans eat a damaging amount of sugar. Let's admit it, most of us also eat too much junk food with little or no nutrition. Doesn't it make good sense to be more selective when it comes to our eating, so we can feel good?

Good health is not only a matter of *what* you eat but *how much* you eat. Overeating is a sin. The Bible calls it gluttony. The simple truth is that when you eat more calories in a day than you burn up in energy, you are adding excessive weight. You do that every day for a month, and you have added ugly, unhealthy pounds. Being overweight damages one's self-image. It cuts one's energy level way down. It is an enemy to good health. It is not new that gluttons have a higher death rate resulting from a variety of diseases caused by their excessive weight. Here is a sobering thought to ponder: with every pound of excessive weight, we shorten our own life expectancy. The Bible has this to say, "For instance, take the matter of eating. God has given us an appetite for food and stomachs to digest it. But that doesn't mean we should eat more than we need . . ." (1 Corinthians 6:13 TLB).

Do you need to lose weight? In spite of hundreds of diets being marketed today, there is basically only one way to properly lose weight. How? By disciplining yourself to eat less food than you burn up in a day. This means deny the lesser (an unbridled appetite) to gain the greater (good health) and all that means for your life. When eating less, make sure that what you eat is high in nutrition.

I am somewhat like the woman who boasted of having lost 200 pounds. When questioned as to her truthfulness, she explained: "Well, actually I lost ten pounds on twenty different occasions." I, too, have indulged in weeks of overeating, then had to diet for months to fit back into my clothes again.

I am trying to accept the fact that I cannot eat everything I want and maintain my present weight. In order to keep my weight where it is, I must sometimes say no to things I would like to say yes to. On other occasions I must say, "Dale, that's enough. Time to stop eating." Few adults can eat everything they want and maintain good weight control. Limit your eating and gain control over your weight.

Principle 2: Shape up With Exercise

Would you agree that our society has a flab problem? The large majority of both men and women are in poor physical condition. When they could be enjoying physical fitness, they are overweight and flabby. Contributing to our delinquency is our modern way of life in which machines do much of the hard work for us.

Where the vast majority of people used to do hard physical labor, many of us do little or no physical work in a day. Throughout history people have walked. Today, we ride.

The problem is that our bodies were designed for physical exertion and do not function well without exercise. Muscles are only kept in tone as they are used. Physical energy is increased through use, while it is decreased by the lack of being used.

Therefore, daily exercise is one activity that you cannot afford to go without. You may choose not to do it, but the results of living with a flabby, out-of-shape body and low energy supply will be anything but rewarding.

There is no other way to keep physically fit except through regular, committed exercise. Gary Mobley found his fortieth birthday to be a miserable experience. Turning forty made him take an honest look in the mirror at himself. When he saw an overweight, sluggish man who could barely make it through a working day, he wasn't very happy with himself. Adding to his bad feeling about himself was the realization that his wife was getting sick and tired of a man who never wanted to do anything except sit down in his easy chair in front of the TV and fall asleep every night.

Gary worked as an accountant in a small accounting firm. His typical day was made up of sitting at a desk pushing a pencil and occasionally answering the phone. About the only time he would get up from his desk was for a break or for lunch.

His body had not always been so flabby and out of shape. In high school and college days he was an outstanding athlete. But through laziness and neglect he had given up physical exercise years before and was, at age forty, reaping an out-of-shape, tired body as a result.

Fortunately for Gary, on his fortieth birthday, he made up his mind that he was going to shape up by committing himself to a daily running program. The very next morning, after his life-changing encounter with himself, Gary put on his tennis shoes and went out running. He hadn't gone very far until he was out of breath and panting as if he were going to die. That night those leg muscles that he hadn't used in a long time let him know that they were still there.

But Gary didn't let aching muscles stop him. The next morning he got up early and went running again. The next day he ran farther. He kept running, gradually increasing both his speed and distance until, three months later, twenty pounds lighter, with his waistline reduced five inches, he felt like a new man. Not only did he look sharp, but his energy level had more than tripled. No longer did he drag through a day but found himself with boundless energy for his wife and family after a hard day's work.

Today Gary is in his mid-fifties and looks like a man ten years younger. He exercises every day and is in top physical condition.

What exercise should a person do? For me it is jogging

every day, the first thing in the morning. For someone else it might be playing tennis three or four times a week. For you, possibly it is calisthenics, swimming, or whatever it is you enjoy doing and will make the commitment to do on a regular, consistent basis.

Once people start regular exercise, what keeps them going is something more than the increased physical capacity they enjoy. As Dr. Kenneth H. Cooper, renowned head of the Aerobics Center in Dallas says, "It's the psychological improvement, the fact that they do feel better. They have a more positive outlook, more enthusiasm and are more productive. A person who is physically fit gains a whole new zest for life that he doesn't have when he's not physically fit."

THE CHOICE IS YOURS—FIT OR FAT.
NO ONE CAN EXERCISE YOUR BODY BUT YOU.
THE THING TO DO IS GET STARTED NOW.

Principle 3: Think Healthy Thoughts

Did you know that how you think affects your health and energy output? Think sick thoughts, and you are going to open up your body to be attacked by a variety of diseases. Think and dwell on something that makes you angry, and your blood pressure is going to go up. Harbor ill feelings toward another person, and you are going to make yourself sick. The Bible says, "As a man thinketh in his heart so is he" (*see* Proverbs 23:7).

Have you ever felt symptoms of being physically ill and gone to the doctor for help and then, after extensive testing and examination, been told you're fine, nothing wrong with you? It's confusing, isn't it? Here you are feeling pain, feeling lousy, and you're told there is nothing to worry about, you're okay.

Once I was having pain in my arms and chest and other parts of my body. This went on for about seven or eight days, and finally Margi made me go to see a doctor. He checked me over carefully. At one point I almost fainted in his office, because I have a very squeamish stomach when it comes to blood and examinations.

I was pretty well convinced that I must be having some trouble with my heart. The symptoms were all there. There have been many heart problems in the history of the Galloway family. The doctor not only examined me thoroughly, but sent me to the cardiac center, where they gave me a thorough testing on the treadmill. When they got all done testing me, there was absolutely nothing wrong with me physically.

I went home concluding that I had made myself sick. For weeks I had been working under heavy stress and had allowed myself to dwell on worry-filled thoughts, and these unhealthy thoughts had made me sick.

The problem of our minds making our bodies sick is much larger than most of us like to admit. As one medical expert has said, "Sickness is not so much an enemy from the outside as it is a breakdown in our internal defenses." Do you know that about 70 to 80 percent of people who go to a doctor, by doctors' own admission, are suffering from emotional and stress-related illnesses caused by unhealthy thoughts? Now they have all the symptoms—headaches, fatigue, ulcers, skin rashes, colitis, arthritis, all the others. They feel pain. They are physically sick. And, with medication they experience temporary relief. But the big question is, how did they get sick? If you trace back to the root cause, 70 percent of the time when we are ill, it is because that we have chosen to think and dwell on unhealthy thoughts.

In a book I read recently under the title *I Know You Hurt but There's Nothing to Bandage,* written by a physician by the name of Donald D. Fisher, I read the true account of a woman by the name of Sylvia who came to see him after five operations. This lady had had five hospitalizations, five surgeries at a total cost of $17,000, to say nothing of the pain incurred, and she still had the original pain in her side. Dr. Fisher explained that when Sylvia came to see him she was having severe diarrhea and a full-blown case of colitis. After having taken her long medical history and learned about all her five operations that did no good in relieving the pain in her side, he took the time to ask her when it all started.

Out came the story that one year before, her pain had started when she went to see her mother who was dying of cancer of the colon. When the doctor asked her where her mother's cancer started, she answered that it was in the bowel and then pointed to the exact spot in her side where her own pain was.

Once it was uncovered that Sylvia's empathy and agony with her own mother's pain were causing her pain in the same spot, it wasn't but two weeks of rest and tranquilizers until she was completely free from the pain.

Next time you are not feeling well, I challenge you to have the courage to ask yourself this penetrating question: *What is making me sick?* Another way to ask it, *Have I been thinking healthy or unhealthy thoughts?* This is a giant step toward enjoying better health. As Carl Rogers, the noted psychologist, said, "Once I accept myself—then I can change." The key concept is *accepting yourself* the way you are. Once you do this, then you can take action to change the way you've been thinking—from negative to positive.

For your own good health the Bible admonishes you to think healthy thoughts when it says, "... Fix your thoughts on what is true and good and right. Think about things that are pure and lovely, and dwell on the fine, good things in others. Think about all you can praise God for and be glad about" (Philippians 4:8 TLB).

I have discovered that, in my own life, when I am eating right, exercising right, and thinking right, it all works together for my good health and high energy level. But to tell you the truth, practicing these three principles that I have shared with you for better health and more energy has not always been easy to do in my life. I love to eat both the wrong things and more than I should eat. I don't always feel like getting out of bed in the morning and going out in the cold rain and jogging. If I were to give in to my lazy side, there are many times that I would just drift along dwelling on unhealthy thoughts.

As I daily work with many people I care so deeply about, I hate to see any of them go on reaping the sick results of an undisciplined life. God has a better way for us to live!

I DARE YOU TO SHAPE UP!

Today I want to rededicate myself in the presence of my Lord Jesus Christ to eat right, exercise daily, and fix my thoughts on healthy thoughts. I have made up my mind I want more out of life than a fat, flabby, tired, sick body and mind that operate at a low energy level. I want, with God's help, to be mentally and physically fit so that I can abound in doing the work of my Lord Jesus. There are many things yet in my life that I want to achieve in Jesus' name. And to do that I must pay the price of disciplining my eating, exercising my body, and choosing and cultivating positive, healthy thoughts.

YOU TOO CAN HAVE BETTER HEALTH AND BOUNDLESS ENERGY IF YOU WILL GET STARTED IN A DAILY LIFE OF DENYING THE LESSER TO GAIN THE GREATER.

Self-evaluation

1. Are you satisfied with your present eating habits?
   If not, for the sake of your good health, what changes do you need to make?
2. Do you consider yourself fit or fat?
   If you are overweight, how many pounds over are you?
3. Write out your own action plan for losing weight.
4. Would you agree that everyone needs an exercise program?
   Do you have a regular exercise program?
   If not, write out an action plan for your own exercise and good health.

5. Have you been thinking healthy thoughts or unhealthy thoughts?

   Write out your own action plan for choosing and cultivating healthy thoughts.

4

Seven Techniques to Control Your Sex Drive

Do you know what is the most popular sport in our world today?

Do you know what is the number-one box-office draw to movies?

Do you know what kind of books and magazines continue to top the best-seller list?

Do you know what a lot of people think about in their leisure time?

Do you know what is as old as Adam and Eve?

Do you know what both young people and old people alike are interested in?

Do you know what first attracts a man to a woman?

The answer to all of these questions is the same three letter word: *sex*. Sex is without a doubt the most popular theme in our world today. Sex is something that everyone has from birth and is interested in until death. The advertisers know this. This is why they use sex to sell us everything from prunes to pencils. Yes—we all have an interest in sex—every one of us. Now I am going to step out in front of the parade of sex and tell you some things that you need to know about sex that our modern society doesn't know.

Who invented sex? Who thought it all up in the first

place? Who in the beginning made male and female? Who first brought Eve to Adam and commanded them, " . . . Be fruitful, and multiply, and replenish the earth" (Genesis 1:28 KJV)? *God did it all.* He is the Originator and Creator of sex. Sex, you might say, is His brainchild.

Sex is one of the beautiful gifts God gives to every person He creates. Just think: You are one of God's special creation, and your sexuality is a sacred gift from the Creator to you.

This may shock some of you. God created all the parts of your human body. That includes your sex organs, with their capacity for enjoyment. A study of the human body points up how wondrously God has designed the male and female sexual parts. What a fabulous job of design and engineering. On the sixth day, having finished all His creation, "And God saw every thing that he had made, and, behold, it was very good . . ." (Genesis 1:31 KJV). God has yet to create anything bad or inferior.

Why did God give to each of us the gift of sex? To bring together male and female in the bond of love and marriage. To experience the mutual joy of oneness. It is God who told us to become "one flesh" (Genesis 2:24 KJV).

Beatrice, a middle-aged woman, said to me, "I thought God created sex for the purpose of propagation of the race." That big word means "bearing children." I said, "Yes, acing to Genesis 1:28 and Psalms 127:3, 4 that is true. But God also created sex for more than propagation. He created it for pleasure." (*See* Proverbs 5:18, 19; Genesis 2:24.) In the Old Testament Book of the Song of Solomon, the ecstasies of lovemaking between a loving husband and a responsive wife are vividly described. How beautiful lovemaking is when carried on as God intended it, under the secure tent of love, commitment and marriage. The marriage act releases daily tensions, fulfills manhood and womanhood, and brings together husband and wife in the blissful experience of oneness. How beautiful it is to completely become each other's as husband and wife in lovemaking.

If you have been prone to feel guilty about your own sexuality—stop it! Start today to thank God for the marvelous way He has made you. Sex, when used as God intended, in the marriage relationship, is a beautiful, enriching experience. The Bible says, speaking of the first man and woman, "And they were both naked, the man and his wife, and were not ashamed" (Genesis 2:25 KJV).

Sex came before sin. Adam and Eve made love before sin entered the garden (*see* Genesis 2:25). *The evil is not in the use of God's good gifts, but in the abuse of them.*

We live in a world that has its mind occupied with the pursuit of pleasure. The time has come for us to remind ourselves of C. S. Lewis's words in his famous *Screwtape Letters:* it is God who "made all the pleasures: all our research so far has not enabled us to produce one." What the devil does is take what God has already created and try to get us to pervert it and misuse it. Sin always diminishes pleasure. If you don't believe that, then why is it that, when people go outside the bounds of marriage for sex, they have to keep increasing the thrill to get the same pleasure return?

The Bible very clearly and repeatedly speaks out forcibly against the misuse and abuse of sex. The Bible minces no words in calling it adultery or fornication. Why does God prohibit sex outside of marriage? For our own good and well-being. History, as well as modern times, depicts repeatedly that there is nothing more destructive and devastating to the human race than sex sins.

As a counselor, I have listened to the heartbreaking consequence of sex sins many times. No two stories, of course, are exactly alike. No two people who have committed sex sins are alike. Some are guilt ridden, some appear not to have much guilt. Some are remorseful, some are defiant. But through all these tangled tales of premarital and extramarital sex adventures runs a thread of disillusionment and destruction. After it is all done, and they are left with nothing but the consequences, they all say the same thing, "It wasn't worth it emotionally or any other way." Someone has said, "Immorality is acute shortsightedness." It seems that they never stop to look ahead—they just plunge in.

A married woman in her late thirties, suffering the guilt-ridden consequence of having had an affair, came to me asking for help. As is often the case, this woman's misuse of sex seemed to be based on resentment she had toward her husband. She wanted to make him pay. "Well, I paid him back," she said. "But I sure paid a price myself. To begin with, I got far more involved with my lover emotionally than he was with me." Then looking right at me she asked pathetically, "Do you realize how humiliating that can be to a woman? Realizing that a man you have given yourself to can slam the door in your face at any moment. Which of course is exactly what happened in the end. In spite of all my tears and pleading, he walked out on me, never to return."

Remorsefully she continued, "Then there are all sorts of dandy little dividends that you never hear about in the magazines and movies. Going in at night and looking at your children asleep in the bed, knowing that one false step on the tightrope and you will damage their lives. Seeing your lover at a party, talking to your husband, and feeling like a dirty cheat." At this point the woman broke down into tears, sobbing over and over, "I hate myself, I hate myself."

And some people want to question why God gave us moral laws? The answer came out of His divine love for us—to spare us the agony and pain that results from sex sins. The wisdom of the Ten Commandments never grows old or out-of-date. It is not repealed because some people choose to abuse and misuse their sex gift.

To you who are suffering the consequences of sex sins, let me say God specializes in new beginnings. If you are like the woman who was taken in an act of adultery, to you Jesus says, ". . . Neither do I condemn thee: go, and sin no more" (John 8:11 KJV). If you need forgiveness, if you need release from the sex sins that have bound you, then ask Jesus to be your Lord and Savior and with His help live a more abundant life and stop abusing your sex gift. Life will work out only one way—that is God's way—He made it like that.

The Bible says, ". . . You must abstain from fornication; each one of you must learn to gain mastery over his body . . ." (1 Thessalonians 4:3, 4 NEB). Again the Bible says, ". . . But sexual sin is never right: our bodies were not made for that, but for the Lord, and the Lord wants to fill our bodies with himself." (1 Corinthians 6:13 TLB). Again and again the Bible warns, admonishes, pleads with and commands us to stay away from damaging sex sins.

Janet was a very attractive counselee, a divorcée in her mid-twenties, who came to see me because her search for the good life had turned into a miserable life.

She told me outright, "These one-night stands have gotten to be one big bore. I've really had it with the whole thing. At first it was fun, I thought. Everybody says that swinging is supposed to be a ball, but believe me, it's not. I have lost all interest in sex. I feel so used and misused. I feel cheap and spent. Worst of all, I've lost my own self-respect."

The other day I was driving down the freeway when I came upon a spot where traffic had slowed up. I wondered what all the hold-up was. Then I saw a male and a female dog mating in the middle of the freeway. I thought, *You know, that's the way dogs are. They do it anywhere, with any dog, at any time. That is a dog's life.*

But God created us for something greater than to live a dog's life. He created us as moral beings with the possibility of living a beautiful life made up of loyalty, commitment, love, and marriage.

In Robert Schuller's classic book *Self-Love, the Dynamic Force of Success,* he shares this story. And although I have read it many years ago I have never forgotten.

A young man shared this story with me. "I was bored one night and went to a neighborhood bar. I met this chick and we started drinking. She was lonely. I was bored. I was unmarried. She was divorced. 'Let's go to Las Vegas,' she suggested. I looked at the hungry invitation in her sultry eyes and immediately put my glass down, paid the bartender, took her arm and headed for the car. She snuggled warmly and hungrily close to me. We roared through the night with visions of a hot bed in a Vegas motel. For some strange reason that I cannot explain, I was suddenly gripped by the thought that this was a pretty cheap thing for me to do. I found myself mentally torn at the sexual compulsion to 'shack-up' with this barfly for whom I had no respect whatsoever. At the same time, glancing at the rear-view mirror, I saw my own eyes. They were the eyes of a potentially wonderful person. I was beginning to feel the disgust and self-loathing that I had known on more than one previous occasion after indulging in a depersonalizing sexual escapade. I pulled over to the shoulder of the road and stopped the car. 'What are you doing?' she asked.

" 'I'm getting out,' I answered abruptly. 'It's your car. Go on to Vegas if you want to. I don't care what you do. I'll thumb a ride back.' I slammed the door shut and watched as she angrily spun the wheels in the gravel and roared furiously away. I stood there alone in the night on a lonely stretch of desert road. Suddenly I felt ten feet tall! I never felt so good in my life! I felt like a triumphant general returning victoriously from a proud battle. That was my moment of self-love."

Controlling your sex drive and living clean morally goes hand in hand with enjoying good feelings about yourself as a person. In other words, you cannot break the moral laws of God and commit sex sins without hurting yourself—to say nothing of the havoc it wreaks in the other party's life or lives.

It is absolutely essential that you take charge of your own sex drive and control it. How well you learn to control your own sex drive will determine whether sex for you is:

Something beautiful or something ugly

Something creative or something destructive

Something that puts the icing on the cake of your marriage or something that tears relationships apart

Something that builds your self-worth or something that destroys your self-respect

It's your sex drive. You can control it, or you can let it get out of control. Both the choice and the results are yours!

A young man who was trying hard to get his messed-up life straightened out asked me, "How do I control my sex drive?" I now share with you the same seven techniques that I shared with this young man.

How to Control Your Sex Drive

TECHNIQUE 1: ACCEPT GOD'S MORAL LAW AS ABSOLUTE AND RIGHT FOR YOURSELF. Look out! The human mind has the amazing ability to rationalize and twist things to fit its own fancy. Many a person never believes in immorality until he decides he would like to try it. The moment you start arguing with the Scriptures and start bending and twisting them to suit yourself, you are headed for trouble. The Bible says, ". . . Make not provision for the flesh, to fulfil the lusts thereof" (Romans 13:14 KJV). On the other hand, the first step in both moral recovery and right control of one's sex gift is to accept what the Scripture says.

There is no excuse for moral flabbiness according to God's holy law. In my experience of counseling I often hear the transgressing mate trying to blame his or her moral failure on the lack of sexual responsiveness in his or her mate.

I'm reminded of what Dr. Richard Taylor, a seminary professor of mine, used to say about this little blame game. He said, "That is a cowardly evasion of moral responsibility." Living clean morally does not depend upon the responsiveness of one's mate. If your mate is warm and responsive to you sexually, then you can be grateful. If not, then draw close to God and appropriate more of His strength and help in your need to master your sex drive. Often in a marriage there are times of physical illness, psychological stress, other events that prevent sexual fulfillment in the way one would desire it. Times like these are opportunities to learn some deep meanings of love.

TECHNIQUE 2: DENY THE LESSER TO GAIN THE GREATER. The sex drive, as strong as it is, is not something that has to overwhelm you. For example you may have an overwhelming desire to swear, but that doesn't mean you have to choose to go ahead and swear. Sex is not like hunger in that you have to satisfy it to go on living. The interesting thing about sexual desire is that it is not long satisfied by one sex act. On the contrary, participation in the sex act often arouses the passion and desire to want more.

Therefore if you do not have the right of sex within a marriage, the way to gain mastery over your sex drive is not by letting it run loose like a wild dog, but by containing it. Contrary to what a lot of pagan philosophies are teaching us today, you do not have to have an active sex life to have a good, happy life. In fact, I have yet to meet a person who had a happy satisfying life as a direct result of having an active sex life only. On the other hand, I have met many contented, happy persons who in their single state have chosen to control and contain their sex drive. So much of the un-happiness and havoc that I see among people are the results of an undisciplined sex life. We need to get it through our heads that as wonderful as sex is there is so much more that goes into making up a good life than sex.

For example, the Apostle Paul gave up both sex and marriage that he might dedicate himself completely to Christian service. He denied the lesser to gain the greater. He learned successfully to subordinate his sex drive. Paul said, "I keep my body under. . . ." (*see* 1 Corinthians 9:27). The big question is, how did he do it? He did it by yielding himself to the Holy Spirit.

TECHNIQUE 3: YIELD YOURSELF TO THE CONTROL OF THE HOLY SPIRIT. The Bible teaches that the most powerful force in all the world is the Holy Spirit. When Jesus was parting from earth, He made it clear that He would not leave us alone or without power. We were not to be orphans. But He would send the Holy Spirit who would come and live within us.

In God's plan *you* are the temple of God.

Haven't you yet learned that your body is the home of the Holy Spirit God gave you, and that he lives within you? Your own body does not belong to you. For God has bought you with a great price. So use every part of your body to give the glory back to God, because he owns it.

1 Corinthians 6:19, 20 TLB

The moment one receives the Lord Jesus Christ as personal Savior, the Holy Spirit comes to live within him. Every Christian has within him the source and the strength, through the Holy Spirit, to control and master sex drives, if he will yield to the Holy Spirit's control.

Yielding is a matter of the will. Victory comes as we pray the same prayer our Lord prayed in the garden, "Not my will but thy will be done." Victory and power to control your sex life will come at the point when you yield your will to domination and control of the Spirit of God, who is now within you.

It is the Holy Spirit that makes us clean and keeps us clean. Give up the control of your own life to the Holy Spirit, who is within you, and you will find the self-control that you need to master your own sex life.

TECHNIQUE 4: REFUSE TO EAT GARBAGE. Someone has said that what goes in is what comes out. In no area is this more true than the area of the mind. What you put into your mind is what you think. And what you think and dwell upon, after a while, is what you become. We are being bombarded in movies, books, and magazines and over our TVs in our homes, with sexual garbage. And the garbage mixture is getting more rotten every day. You cannot keep on eating garbage without having it make you morally sick. Part of what we are being fed is so subtle, while some of it is straightforward hard-core.

The point is, if we are not selective with what we read and see, then we are going to be eating a lot of garbage. And if we eat a lot of garbage, we are going to become morally sick. Who would eat food that had turned rotten? Certainly not anyone in charge of his own mind. What you and I have got to do is take charge of our own minds. We must use our selection processes, have the good sense to stand up and say,

"No, I am not going to feed myself that immoral garbage anymore."

TECHNIQUE 5: DISCIPLINE YOUR SEX THOUGHTS. Listen in on an idle conversation between non-Christian men. The chances are that a large portion of it will revolve around sex jokes punctuated by four-letter words. When a man becomes a Christian, he becomes a brand new person, and the Holy Spirit begins to talk to him about changing both his language and his thought patterns. Jesus knew the danger of lust when He said, "I say unto you That whosoever looketh on a woman to lust after her has committed adultery with her already in his heart" (Matthew 5:28 KJV).

What should a man do when lustful thoughts come into his mind? A good policy to follow is: don't take the second look. The first look may be beyond your control, but you have the power to turn your head the other way. When a lustful thought comes into your mind, take charge and do not allow yourself to dwell upon it. A good way to do this is to redirect your thinking onto something else.

The Apostle Paul said to the young man Timothy, "Run from anything that gives you the evil thoughts that young men often have, but stay close to anything that makes you want to do right . . ." (2 Timothy 2:22 TLB).

Be brutally frank and honest with yourself. Don't play games or try to kid yourself; when you find that you are attracted to another person sexually, stay away from it. Watch out for low times emotionally. Those are the moments when we are often tempted the most to escape into the loony land of sexual exploration. Don't do anything when you are feeling bad that you wouldn't do when you are feeling good.

Don't compromise yourself with sin at any point. To do so is to lose spiritual power and victory in your life. To do so is to settle for an inferior life-style. The story goes that a robin was offered a worm for a feather. The bird thought that this was a good bargain—it would save a lot of hunting for worms, and he would not miss a feather. But one dreadful day the robin awoke to the fact that his feathers were gone, and he could not fly. He had sold his power to fly for worms. He was earthbound.

People sell out their greatness for such trivial things. God created you to live with dignity. To be a person of worth and value, He calls you to live clean in an unclean world. Step out from the crowd and be the special person God wants you to be.

TECHNIQUE 6: FLEE FROM SEX SINS.   Joseph was a hand-some, healthy young Hebrew man. When Joseph arrived in Egypt as a slave, he was purchased by Potiphar, who was captain of the king's bodyguards. The Lord greatly blessed Joseph in the home of his master, so that everything he did succeeded. Potiphar was so pleased with Joseph and with his special ability that he put him in charge of all his household and business affairs.

Potiphar had a wife who was typical of so much of our society today. She was shameless, accommodating, without loyalty, selfish, and living life on the low, fleshly level. She was not much more than an animal in the pursuit of her passions. She set out to lure Joseph into committing an im-moral act with her. She tantalized him and then finally openly invited him to come take her to bed.

Joseph, as a man of God, lived life on a higher level.

Things like honesty, loyalty, righteousness, reason, and putting God first meant more to Joseph than a fleeting moment of immorality. He said to her, ". . . How can I do such a wicked thing as this? It would be a great sin against God" (Genesis 39:9 TLB).

We read in the Bible how she persistently tried to drag him down to her level, day after day. Then one day as he was in the house, doing his work—no one else was around—"She came and grabbed him by the sleeve demanding, 'Sleep with me.' He tore himself away, but as he did his jacket slipped off and she was left holding it as he fled the house" (Genesis 39:12 TLB). Joseph fled as fast as he could go. There comes a time as you and I live in this unclean world that if we are going to live clean, we are going to have to run as fast as we can to get away from evil.

The Bible directly tells us, ". . . Run from sex sin. No other sin affects the body as this one does. When you sin this sin it is against your own body" (1 Corinthians 6:18 TLB, *see also* 1 Timothy 6:11).

TECHNIQUE 7: SAVE YOUR SEX GIFT FOR YOUR MARRIAGE PARTNER.   Sex, love, and marriage all belong together. Marriage is like a tent that covers the act of sex. Marriage gives sex a security it must have to be at its best. What is a woman's greatest need? To feel protected and secure. Outside the marriage tent there is no way a woman can feel secure in her sex and love. Marriage gives sex the commitment that it must have to be responsible and mutually fulfilling.

Let yourself go. The Bible says, "Marriage is honourable in all, and the bed undefiled . . ." (Hebrews 13:4 KJV). Sexual relations, sexual intercourse at the right time, the right place, with your mate, is just beautiful! *This is good.*

The Scriptures teach us that we are not to withhold our bodies from our mates. In fact it tells us that our bodies belong to our mates. This rules out things like emotional blackmail. To withhold or reward sexually to get one's own way is wrong. It is to misuse the sacred gift of sex and to hurt the free-flowing spirit of love and sex in your marriage (*see* 1 Corinthians 7:2–9).

Today the argument is given by those who would have us all live a dog's life that to be sexually promiscuous is to be better prepared to have a rich sex life in marriage. This is the devil's lie. We who counsel with people see firsthand how sexual promiscuity opens Pandora's box. How many times I have worked with persons having difficulty with sex in their marriage because of guilt from sex acts participated in outside of their marriage vows. To be sexually promiscuous is to become susceptible forever to the devastation of flashback comparison.

It seems to me that to withhold oneself until marriage is to be like a runner on the starting line waiting for the gun to sound. When the gun goes off, you're ready to spring ahead, giving the race your best and putting your all into it. Wise indeed is the man or woman who saves the precious sex gift for marriage, then gives it all fully and completely to his or her beloved.

TO MAKE THE BEST USE OF YOUR SEX GIFT, DENY THE LESSER TO GAIN THE GREATER.

CHAPTER 5

Understanding and Learning How to Handle Your Anger

Do you think Christian authors ever get mad?
Do you think I ever get angry?
Do you ever get angry?

LET'S FACE the truth: Like it or not, anger is a common emotion to every member of the human race. Every normal person, be he a committed Christian or not, experiences the fiery emotion of anger. Anger may be understood as a stirred-up feeling of displeasure. Often it is accompanied by feelings of having been in some way mistreated. It is also true that any feeling of frustration usually gives rise to anger.

As natural as it is for each of us to experience the emotion of anger in our daily life, learning to control it is not an option but a must. Runaway anger is like a raging sea that destroys anything and everything that gets in its way. To be out of control emotionally is always dangerous, and doubly so when the emotion out of control is anger.

Just recently I received this testimonial from a viewer of our New Hope television program after I had spoken on the subject of how to handle your anger.

Said the man that I'll call Matt, "When I get angry, I feel like killing. I find it hard to believe, but recently in a blind rage I almost killed one of my friends. I don't know what came over me, but afterwards I couldn't believe that I had kicked him in the face again and again, trying to kill him. Lord help me, if it hadn't have been for some bystanders pulling me off him, I would have committed murder. It all happened when I allowed my temper to get the best of me."

In Topeka, Kansas, an angry insurance agent, who should have known better, after a furious quarrel with his wife, dashed out to his car, angrily yelling, "You may never see me again."

His words proved to be prophetic. A few minutes later, recklessly speeding down the highway, driven by an uncontrollable rage, he ran head-on into a truck and was instantly killed.

Researchers who have interviewed countless families of persons who have died at the wheel in car accidents have discovered that half of these have serious personal conflicts in the hours preceding their death. Anger is a killer, on the highway, that is second only to alcoholism.

Yesterday I was counseling with a couple who needed my help, but we were getting nowhere. We were wasting their time and my time. What was wrong? The problem was that the young man who wouldn't admit to having anger was so full of it that his overheated emotions made it impossible to have any meaningful dialogue together.

Confronting him in all honesty concerning his anger, I expressed to him that I hoped he wouldn't do anything to harm his wife physically after leaving the appointment. It was not that he was a violent person, because I had known him to be a gentle man, but in his state of uncontrolled anger, I couldn't predict what would happen.

He assured me that he wouldn't do anything to hurt another person physically, but at the same time was blinded to how destructive his uncontrolled anger was to both his physical health and to his relationships, beginning with those closest to him.

Anger is the one emotion that no one can afford to let go uncontrolled, simply because runaway anger is always destructive. It can tear your relationships apart faster than you can, in your rational times, work to rebuild them.

One of man's greatest needs today is to learn to understand the power of anger and to learn, with God's help, how to control it. The Bible says, "It is better to be slow-tempered than famous; it is better to have self-control than to control an army." (Proverbs 16:32 TLB).

Truth You Need to Know About Anger

UNDERSTAND AND RECOGNIZE THAT ANGER IS A NORMAL EMOTION. It is a God-given emotion. As we live our lives there are going to be happenings and circumstances which cause us to feel the strong emotion of anger. Experiencing the emotion by itself is not sin. The Bible says, "Be angry and sin not . . ." (*see* Ephesians 4:26).

Anger by itself is neither good nor evil. Contrary to what some people have mistakenly been taught, to feel anger is not the same as to sin. According to the teachings of the Bible, it is how a person handles or mishandles his anger that determines the right and wrong of it.

And surprising as it may be to some Christians, there are times where anger can be used in a positive way. For example, someone says to me, "It cannot be done." That is usually enough to stir the strong emotion of anger within me, to spur me on to accomplish the impossible feat. There are some things that we need to get stirred up about.

All around us are the flagrant breaking of God's laws, injustice, and wrongdoing. The Old Testament prophet Amos was an example of one who in his rage cried out against evil when he said, ". . . Let justice roll down like waters, and righteousness like an ever-flowing stream" (Amos 5:24 RSV). It would do most Christians good to get a little more stirred up over the evil that's present in our world.

We see a classic example in the Scriptures of Jesus getting stirred up to the point of anger and acting out that anger in a right way. Filled with concern for God's House:

> Jesus made a whip from some ropes and chased them all out, and drove out the sheep and oxen, scattering the money changers' coins over the floor and turning over their tables! Then, going over to the men selling doves, he told them, "Get these things out of here. Don't turn my Father's House into a market!"
>
> John 2:15, 16 TLB

There is a right time and place to speak out a stirred-up concern for what is right.

A sincere woman wanted to know, "Pastor, when does anger become sin?" My reply: "Whenever it becomes destructive."

Two Ways People Mishandle Their Anger

THE FIRST WRONG WAY TO HANDLE ANGER IS TO TAKE IT OUT ON SOMEONE ELSE.   To hurt or harm another individual is sin. To blow your top and shout at someone else is not to be wise, but to be a fool, according to Scriptures. (*See* Proverbs 29:11.)

To take your anger out on another person is:

Not healthy, but unhealthy
Not the solution to problems, but the compounder of problems
Not the builder of love, but the destroyer of love
Not the healer of relationships, but the damager of relationships

A very important part of learning to live the superior Christian life of self-discipline is to learn to stop taking your anger out on those closest to you. The Scriptures teach,

Stop being mean, bad-tempered and angry. Quarrelling, harsh words, and dislike of others should have no place in your lives. Instead, be kind to each other, tenderhearted, forgiving one another, just as God has forgiven you because you belong to Christ.

Ephesians 4:31, 32 TLB

THE SECOND COMMON WAY THAT PEOPLE MISHANDLE THEIR ANGER IS TO SUPPRESS IT. This common practice is disease producing and is downright unhealthy. To bottle up unresolved anger on the inside is a very unhealthy thing to do. Suppressed anger hurts and keeps on hurting. Unfortunately, many very fine Christian people wrongly deal with their emotion of anger by trying to deny it. You may choose to deny it, but if it is there, it is going to keep on hurting you deep down inside. As the famous writer John Powell says, "When I suppress my emotion, my stomach keeps score."

And when it gets to a certain number, it's going to make you ill in one way or another.

Suppressed anger is like a jack-in-the-box. It always has a way of popping out at some unguarded moment. Have you ever had the experience of making a critical or sarcastic remark about another person and being surprised at what you said? What was happening was that your anger was slipping out in an unguarded moment and expressing itself.

The husband who is angry at his wife for not meeting his sexual needs may surprise himself by making cutting little remarks in front of other people. You know those little comments that are supposed to be funny but really aren't. They're cutting, and they cause the other person to be wounded in his or her spirit.

Now if you can't take it out on another person, and you can't bury it down inside, what are you going to do with your anger? One thing for certain: What you choose to do with it will make the difference between sickness and health, turmoil and peace, broken relationships and harmonious relationships, senseless destruction and constructive debate.

As a boy I grew up in Columbus, Ohio, and revelled in the exciting football tradition of Ohio State University. After all these years I'm still an Ohio State fan.

It was a sad day for Ohio State fans when, on national television, one of the winningest coaches in the history of college football and a veteran of twenty-eight years at Ohio State, Woody Hayes, in a fit of rage disgraced himself and his fans by slugging his way out of a job.

We happened to be sitting at home in Portland, Oregon, watching the Gator Bowl on December twenty-ninth, when it happened. In a final uncontrolled act of frustration over a season of intercepted passes, Woody Hayes hit a Clemson player who had just picked off a last-ditch Art Schlictar pass, assuring Ohio State's Gator Bowl defeat. I saw it, but until the instant replay, I didn't believe my own eyes.

Here was this great coach of thirty-three seasons, who stood at the very top of coaches in American football history, losing control completely and hitting a player on another team. Well, it cost Woody his job, and worse than that, it ended his long, illustrious career on a very sour note.

Woody Hayes is not the only one who has been hurt by failing to control his anger. Control is a need in each of our lives. The man or woman who has control over anger has a great advantage in every area of life.

Good news! With Christ's help you do not have to be manhandled by your own runaway anger, but you can learn how to control your anger.

To Handle Your Anger in a Healthy Way, Practice These Nine Principles

1. CONFESS IT. The only healthy way to handle anger is not to blow your top or suppress it. The healthy way to handle anger is to confess it. There is no better way to handle anger.

Unfortunately, a lot of people are not in touch with their own emotions. Chris's love for Michael appeared to be either dormant or all wiped out. In a counseling session she told me that Michael's anger had destroyed her love. She described him as being a very angry young man.

A few days later, when I had my session with Michael, I asked him if he ever got angry at his wife. To him I said, "From what your wife has told me I know that you don't beat her, and being a Christian you don't swear at her, but tell me, what do you do when you have strong feelings of displeasure inside toward her?"

Shrugging his shoulders as if it were no big deal, he said, "Oh, I just don't talk to her for a week." The tragedy was that he was blindly unaware of his silent treatment as being destructive anger. Without realizing it, with his silent sulking he was saying to his wife, "You are not worth talking to." Aware or not, ten years of silent anger had devastated this marriage almost beyond repair.

The first step in learning how to handle your anger is to become aware of your own emotion by asking yourself: *What am I feeling?*

Whenever you feel abused, misused, frustrated, despised, scorned, cursed, humiliated, shamed, unjustly criticized, taken advantage of, unfairly bawled out, irritated, beat up, stepped on, brutalized, betrayed, and unappreciated, you can expect to have some feelings of anger.

When you're angry, do yourself a favor: admit it. Everyone experiences anger, but it is only those who have the openness to admit their anger and confess it who learn how to handle it in positive ways.

It is a crying shame, the number of Christian people who have mistakenly made it a habit to hide their anger and who, as a result, suffer the unhealthy consequences. It is important to understand that a Christian is not one who is perfect in behavior but is one who is learning how to live Christ's superior way. Learn to confess your anger and you have taken a big step on the road to learning how to control your anger.

2. TRACE THE CAUSE OF YOUR ANGER. Often my wife, Margi, and I will have people into our home for special sharing and instruction in preparation for membership into our church. A couple of months ago, just a few minutes before a couple of dozen class members arrived, I got so mad that I thought I was going to pop a blood vessel.

What terrible timing! Here we were preparing to instruct people in the abundant life that Jesus came to give us, and I was consumed with anger.

I hate to tell you who was the target of my anger. It was the person I love the most, Margi. Let me be quick to tell you that I didn't hit her or even speak a mean word to her. I just gave her my specially designed dirty look. By this non-verbal display of anger, I deeply wounded her spirit.

Needless to say, I was not at my best in teaching the class that evening, for the simple reason that I yet had to deal with my own anger. After the people left that night, I traced my anger to the root cause. I discovered that I had become angry because I felt blocked in the goal I was trying to achieve. What actually happened was that I had asked Margi to do something that I thought was important. I wanted it done immediately, and she was busy doing what she thought was important.

Now understanding what had caused my anger, I was able to deal with it by confessing my anger to Margi and asking her to forgive me. Graciously she forgave me, and her wounded spirit was healed, and we kissed and made up.

Next time you start to feel that stirring emotion of anger, ask yourself this question: *Why am I angry?* Keep asking yourself that question until you trace the cause of your anger. It is often helpful, when tracing the cause of your anger, to talk it out with a close friend or counselor.

A good learning exercise in tracing your anger is to take time to write down the things that you recognize that from time to time cause you to feel the emotion of anger.

When I took the time to do this for myself, I discovered that the following things caused me to feel the emotion of anger:

Being taken advantage of by someone else

Suffering unfair treatment

Having a legitimate demand go unmet

Having my worth not recognized

Being shown up in front of people whom I want to think well of me

Having someone stand in the way of a goal I am trying to achieve

Having expectations that are not fulfilled

Being unable to control persons or situations that I want to control

Having another person being uninterested in what I have to say

Being taken for granted

As you do this valuable exercise you will gain understanding that will aid you in learning to control this powerful emotion.

3. ACCEPT PERSONAL RESPONSIBILITY FOR YOUR ANGER.
The other day someone did something, and I got stirred
up inside and said, "He made me so mad." Chances are,
you, too, have made this same statement. I ask you, is that
a true statement? Can another person make you or me
mad?

The truth is, no one can make another person mad unless
that person chooses to be mad. No one can make you lose
control of your emotions except you. You choose. The
choice is yours.

When we become angry and mishandle our emotions, we
have no one to blame but ourselves.

NO ONE IS RESPONSIBLE FOR YOUR ANGER BUT YOU.

A giant step toward becoming a mature person in handling your anger is to stop blaming others, to stop copping
out, and to accept responsibility for your own emotional reaction of anger. The truth is, you are the only one who can
deal with your anger.

4. TRAIN YOURSELF TO HOLD YOUR TONGUE UNTIL YOU
COOL DOWN. If you speak before you cool down your
emotions, you are going to be sorry.

The more emotions heat up, the more reason goes out the
window. The Bible says, "A wise man controls his temper.
He knows that anger causes mistakes" (Proverbs 14:29 TLB).
When you're angry, you can go ahead and blow your top if

you want to, but such action is not wise, but foolish. Instead of solving problems, it only compounds them and makes matters far worse. The Bible says, "A hot-tempered man starts fights and gets into all kinds of trouble" (Proverbs 29:22 TLB).

The woman asked, "How do you keep from blowing your top and making things worse?" I suggested to her, "The next time you start boiling inside, count to ten before you speak. Or do as one woman discovered she could do to cool her anger. Repeat the first ten words of the Lord's Prayer over and over: "Our Father who art in heaven, Hallowed be thy name. . . ."

Discipline yourself to cool down before you speak, and you will be the winner. The Bible says, "A soft answer turns away wrath, but a harsh word stirs up anger" (Proverbs 15:1 RSV). When the conflict is happening, back off, cool down, gain your composure, then speak softly, and you will be a peacemaker instead of a troublemaker.

5. WORK OUT YOUR AGGRESSION IN A HEALTHY WAY. I have personally discovered that when I have a lot of pent-up feelings inside, if I go play a competitive game of tennis, it works wonders for me. I can just hit that old ball as hard as I want. For me it is a positive way of working out my aggressions as well as being a sport I really enjoy.

I've heard of people who work out their aggressions by chopping wood, digging in the flower beds, mowing the grass, working at a hobby, jogging, and a variety of other physical exercises.

If nothing else, buy yourself a punching bag. Far better to punch out the bag—that is the punching bag—than to make one of your loved ones the old bag and punch him out with your anger. Any time and any way that you can work out your anger in a positive way, it is the healthy thing for you to do. An added benefit is that the people closest to you are going to be a whole lot happier, because you are going to be easier to live with.

6. GAIN SELF-CONTROL BY LOSING CONTROL TO THE HOLY SPIRIT. Two cars are driving down the highway. One is an ambulance on an errand of mercy, saving a life by taking someone to needed medical help. The other car is a late-model sedan, but it swerves recklessly around the curves and finally, while attempting to pass another car, causes a terrible head-on collision in which three people are killed.

What is the difference between these two cars and their behavior? The motor? The type of body? No! There is one main difference: who is in the driver's seat. One was a man on an errand of mercy, the other a drunken driver. In our emotional life it makes a great deal of difference who is in the driver's seat—self or Christ. It is through giving up the control of our own lives to Christ that we gain the power of the Holy Spirit within us that gives us self-control.

In the Scriptures we are commanded, "And be not drunk with wine, wherein is excess; but be filled with the Spirit" (Ephesians 5:18 KJV). This is exactly what will give us the power to control our emotions that we do not as yet have mastery over.

One of the fruits of the Spirit listed in Galatians 5:22 is "self-control." I remember well as a teenager that I had such an uncontrollable temper that it often hurled me into a fight before I knew what was happening to me. People who know me today see me as a leader who has his emotions under control. I have come a long way since the days when I was a hot-tempered teenager.

What has made the difference in my life and many others? The difference is that at fifteen years of age I not only received Jesus Christ as my Savior, but I surrendered myself to the filling of the Holy Spirit. I put Jesus in the driver's seat of my total life, which includes my emotions. Giving up to Him my life that was out of control, He has given back to me a new self-control.

I discovered that as I live in the Spirit, the fruits of the Spirit evidence themselves in my life. The more we yield ourselves to the Holy Spirit's control, the more power He gives us to control our emotional lives. *Let Him have His way with you.* Not in part, but totally.

7. DON'T NURSE A GRUDGE.   One thing about anger, the longer you hold onto it, the more it gets a hold on you. The longer you allow it to be within you, the deeper it goes down into your being. Nursing a grudge can grow into a consuming hate.

The Bible advises, "If you are angry, don't sin by nursing your grudge. Don't let the sun go down with you still angry—get over it quickly, for when you are angry you give a mighty foothold to the devil" (Ephesians 4:26, 27 TLB).

When your feelings are hurt, deal with it quickly. The quicker you get it straightened out, the sooner you are going to feel better. Don't keep sulking and licking your wounds. Let ill feelings have no overnight lodging. One of the best pieces of advice that can be given to newlyweds is this: make up before going to bed. In other words, don't take ill feelings into your sleep. If you do, they will work on you in a negative way.

What we need to do is to learn to treat our emotional wounds as quickly as we would treat physical wounds. When you are injured physically, do you wait a week before taking care of the wounds? Certainly not! Why not? Because to wait to treat the wound is to compound the injury. The same thing is true emotionally.

The rule is to wait only long enough to cool down, then deal with it quickly, honestly, and openly.

8. BE OPEN AND HONEST WITH THE OTHER PERSON ABOUT WHAT IS STIRRING YOU UP.   A stepmother relates this experience that happened in her life. "When a teenage stepchild came for a summer visit, she went out one night without telling us where she was going. Upon her return she was stunned when I blew up, for I was really angry and said some reactionary things that surprised me. After all, all she had done was to take a walk down to the corner store.

"Later, after she had gone to bed, I tried to see why I had become so upset and unreasonable. I discovered that there had been a whole series of irritations since her arrival that I had passed off as being too small to make waves about. This last incident was the one too many that exploded the sticks of dynamite that I had been storing up inside. These things had gotten all blown out of proportion because I had not been honest with her about the things that were bothering me. The next day I told her what I had seen about myself, where I had been wrong in taking my anger out on her, and I asked her for forgiveness.

"After she had forgiven me for my outburst of anger, I

was able to share with her the little annoyances that were bothering me, like her clothes being left on the floor in the bedroom. She saw how thoughtless she had been and apologized, and we both felt closer to each other than ever."

The important principle is that before we can talk about what someone is doing that is bothering us, we must first deal with our own anger. If we don't do this, then it will come out the wrong way and cause additional misunderstanding and suffering.

First, deal with your own anger by confessing it openly. Whatever you do, don't say, "You're making me angry." That will put the other person on the defensive for sure. Better to say something like, "I'm feeling angry, and I am sorry." Having confessed your own anger and dealing with it, you are now ready to talk about the things that are bothering you. Speak the truth always, but do it in love. Do not exaggerate. (*See* Ephesians 4:15, 25.)

9. SET YOUR SPIRIT FREE BY PRAYING FOR THE PERSON WHO HAS INJURED YOU. Prayer works wonders when you work at it. When it comes to praying for someone who has done you wrong, prayer isn't always easy. But do it anyway. And as you do pray for that person who has injured you the most amazing thing will happen. Your anger will be replaced with understanding and love. Make these words a part of your prayer, "Jesus, fill my heart with a new understanding and overflowing love. Take away the ill feelings and make me clean through and through."

FOR THE GREATEST CONTROL POSSIBLE—LET JESUS CONTROL YOU—ALL OF YOU. NOT JUST FOR A DAY—BUT EVERY DAY.

"O TO BE LIKE THEE,
 O TO BE LIKE THEE,
 BLESSED REDEEMER, PURE AS THOU ART
 COME IN THY SWEETNESS
 COME IN THY FULLNESS:
 STAMP THINE OWN IMAGE
  DEEP ON MY HEART."

THOMAS O. CHISHOLM

DENY UNCONTROLLED ANGER
AND
GAIN SELF-CONTROL.

Self-evaluation

1. When was the last time you experienced anger?

2. How did you handle it? Did you blow up? Did you suppress it? Did you confess it?

3. What caused your anger?

4. At what point did you become aware that you were angry?
   Before or after the fact?

5. Grade yourself from A to F on the following ways of handling anger:

   (A) Excellent (B) Very good (C) Fair (D) Poor (F) Failing
   _____ 1. Confess it.
   _____ 2. Trace the cause of your anger.

_____ 3. Accept personal responsibility for your anger.

_____ 4. Train yourself to hold your tongue until you cool down.

_____ 5. Work out your aggression in a healthy way.

_____ 6. Gain self-control by losing control to the Holy Spirit.

_____ 7. Don't nurse a grudge.

_____ 8. Be open and honest with the other person about what is stirring you up.

_____ 9. Set your spirit free by praying for the person who has injured you.

CHAPTER 6

Eight Steps to Mastering Your Moods

When they were up they were up,
And when they were down they were down;
And when they were only half-way up,
They were neither up nor down.

THIS LITTLE POEM was a description given to the Duke of York's ten thousand men. It could well be the description of scores of people who have not yet learned how to master their moods.

When I was a teenager, growing up in Columbus, Ohio, quite often on a hot summer night four or five of us boys would pile in an old jalopy and head for Buckeye Lake. Buckeye Lake is an amusement park in central Ohio. We went there to look at the girls and ride the roller coaster.

I vividly remember how riding the roller coaster was like climbing inside of a yo-yo and being thrown up and down. Once you were aboard and it had started, there was no way to escape until it came to the end of the track. While riding, one moment you were up and thrilled, and the next breath you were scared to death. Up, up, up the roller coaster would take you, and then suddenly it would hurl you down,

down, down at a lightning speed that made your stomach feel like the very bottom of it was going to drop out.

Riding the roller coaster is supposed to be a fun high, yet from my experience, all the time I was riding it I was holding on for dear life and secretly begging the crazy monster to please stop. There are a lot of people who live their lives on an emotional roller coaster and would like to get off the crazy monster.

A bright young man who was plagued half the time by depression asked me this question. "What can I do to get on top of my bad moods?" A struggling housewife wanted to know, "How do I get victory over my low mood swings?" An executive secretary confided to a friend, "I like my boss a whole lot, except the days that my boss is in a bad mood. Then my job becomes almost unbearable."

As spring follows winter and fall comes after summer, so our moods change. It is one of the realities of life that each day I awaken with moods that have changed from yesterday. Individuals seem to have one of two mood patterns. The first mood pattern is what I call the Rocky Mountain high, Grand Canyon low pattern. The people who have this mood pattern swing extremely high, and then they go lower than a mole. The second mood pattern is more like the small rolling hills I used to see as a boy in southern Ohio. The people who follow this pattern in daily life are a little bit up and then a little bit down. They have the good fortune of avoiding the extremes. Which of these two mood patterns best represents yours?

Whichever one of these two mood patterns best describes your natural mood flow, there is a more satisfying, enriching life awaiting you as you dare to use positive self-discipline in mastering your own moods.

Did you hear about the six men who went mountain climbing? They had just scaled their way to the top when one of the men fell over a cliff into a crevasse. His companion climbers tried to rescue him. Ever so carefully they leaned over the cliff and yelled, "Joe, Joe, Joe, are you all right?" Back came Joe's voice, "I'm alive, I'm alive, . . . but I think both my arms are broken."

"We will toss a rope down to you and pull you up," yelled the rescuers. "Hurry, please hurry!" cried Joe.

Within a few minutes the men began to pull Joe up. When they had him about three-fourths of the way up, it suddenly dawned on them that Joe had said he had broken both his arms. "Joe," one of them yelled, "if you broke both of your arms, how are you holding on?" Joe responded, "With my teeeeeeeeeeth!"

How many times have you felt you were at the end of your rope, just barely holding on with your teeth and feeling so low that they would have to use a jack to get you off the ground? There are those times in each of our lives when we feel lower than a mole. At that moment, the desire for living is not all that great.

How do you get up when you're down? Begin by acknowledging and accepting that you are in an emotional downer. It's a normal happening from time to time in every person's life. Next, try to trace down the cause of your depressed feelings. Do this by talking it out with a friend or praying it out with your Heavenly Father, or even better, both. Having done this, make up your mind that you are not going to be beaten by a downer, but with Christ's help, you are going to rise up.

How can you get on top of your moods? How can you master your own moods?

Take These Eight Steps to Mastering Your Moods

1. DEVELOP UNDERSTANDING OF YOUR OWN MOOD CHANGES. Spend some important self-improvement time analyzing your moods. Whenever you find that you are touchy, hard to get along with, full of negative emotions like fear, worry, anxiety, ask yourself why. Possibly it is because you have been listening to negative thinkers; you're worried about a problem; you're harboring an ill feeling toward someone else; or there is a chemical imbalance in your body. Once you have traced down the cause or causes of your bad mood, then you can begin to take the needed steps to correct it.

Sometimes a physical condition is the cause for sagging emotions. A chemical imbalance within the body can play havoc with our emotions. The kinds of food and amounts we eat have a direct effect on our moods. Physical illness has a direct bearing on our moods. If you ever experience any prolonged depression contrary to your usual mood pattern, then you should, by all means, consult your family doctor.

An ill spirit within can cut you down emotionally. A man whom we will call Philip was terribly depressed. His low mood had caused him to separate from his wife. After Philip had been sharing with Jerry for several days, Jerry called my office and made arrangements for his friend to come and see me.

Philip's opening words to me after we had greeted each other were these: "I don't love my wife anymore." As Philip shared with me I sensed he had a deep desire to serve God and do what was right by his family but was really being torn apart by the negative feelings that had seized control of his life.

What do you do when you don't feel like you love your mate anymore, especially when you are supposed to be a committed Christian and committed to living according to God's family plan in the Bible?

One of the things that I have learned across the years from working with fellow human beings is that the true cause of the problem is often far below the surface.

As this sincere man shared, it became clear to me that he was filled with years of resentments toward his wife. In the spirit of Jesus' love I began to help Philip to see his resentments and that resentment is a sin. I taught him that he was not responsible for his wife's attitudes and actions, but that he was responsible to God for his own ill feeling. That whatever else he did, whether or not he went back to his wife, for his own well-being, he had to deal with this ill feeling that was dragging him down on the inside.

RESENTMENT TOWARD ANOTHER PERSON WILL DRAG YOU DOWN EMOTIONALLY.

I gave Philip an exercise to do. I got him to commit that he would go to the apartment where he was living alone and write down on a piece of paper everything he resented his wife for. Then he would take that piece of paper and give it to God. It was Friday afternoon when Philip left my office.

I hadn't been in my office very long Monday morning before Philip called me up. There was a newfound joy in his voice. Excitedly he related his freeing experience.

He said, "When I left your office I went right home, and I began writing all the resentments down that I had for my wife. It got pretty heavy. I didn't know all the deep resentments that I had buried in there for the past years. After I had finished writing and crying out all the resentments, in a step of faith I burned up the paper and gave it to God. Even as the paper was burning, a miracle began to take place, and those resentments went away. As amazing as it is, I found myself loving my wife in a new, fresh way." Philip climaxed his overflowing report by telling me how good it felt to be back home with his wonderful wife.

A week later I talked to Philip again, and he related to me that now he could not even remember the reasons he had had for resenting his wife. Coming clean with God had worked wonders for him. (*See* 1 John 1:9.)

If you are being dragged down emotionally by an ill spirit, I challenge you in the name and power of Jesus Christ to open up and pour out all those destructive feelings to God. Confess and ask Him to cleanse you and make you whole. In His presence get out all the rubbish and let Him make you clean through and through. Even as you do this, believe it—there is flowing into your life love, peace and the lifting emotion of joy.

A study of the Bible reveals that some pretty big spiritual giants suffer from low mood swings. Shortly after experiencing one of the greatest answers to prayer in history,

Elijah's emotional bottom dropped out, and he sat down under a juniper tree, "... and he requested for himself that he might die...." (1 Kings 19:4 KJV).

In the midst of great suffering, a discouraged Job said, "My soul is weary of my life ..." (Job 10:1 KJV). David, who had a very positive personality and wrote most of the Psalms of praise, knew what it was to have a low mood swing. On one occasion he shared his feeling when he said, "... My soul is cast down within me ..." (Psalms 42:6 KJV). Jeremiah, one of the major prophets, who spoke with holy boldness, in a moment of extreme loneliness and self-pity said, "Woe is me ..." (Jeremiah 15:10 KJV).

Understand that having a low mood does not mean that you are not a Christian. But it does mean that your mood is in a downswing. Remember, the tide goes out, and the tide comes in. When your tide's out emotionally, draw close to the Lord and let His strength cover your weakness. I love this promise from the Bible, "But they that wait upon the Lord shall renew their strength; they shall mount up with wings as eagles; they shall run, and not be weary; and they shall walk, and not faint" (Isaiah 40:31 KJV).

2. ACCEPT PERSONAL RESPONSIBILITY FOR YOUR OWN MOODS. To blame a bad mood on other people is to fail to deal with reality. Now it's true that other people do affect our moods, but they cannot cause our moods unless we allow them to. The power of choice is ours. What takes place on the inside of us is our own responsibility to work with and to bring under control. No one can get you in or out of a bad mood but you.

What excuse is there for taking a bad mood out on other people? There is none. To take your bad mood out on others is to sin against them.

What you give is what you get. My good friend Dr. Robert Schuller likes to tell the story about a mother who disciplines her son for his behavior. The boy doesn't say anything to her; he knows better. But the first chance he gets he goes out the back door and runs off into the woods. There, out of earshot of his mother, he yells at the top of his voice, "I hate you, I hate you, I hate you." Back comes the echo through the woods, "I hate you, I hate you, I hate you." The voice echoing the ugly words scares the boy and he runs home as fast as his legs will carry him. Once safely inside, still panting he exclaims, "Mother, mother, there is a strange man out in the woods and he is yelling 'I hate you, I hate you, I hate you.' "

The wise mother takes the little boy by the hand, leads him back up into the woods. Then she says to her son, "Now I want you to say as loudly as you can three times, 'I love you.' " Feeling safe with his mother nearby, the boy yells, "I love you, I love you, I love you." Back come the beautiful words, "I love you, I love you, I love you." Concludes my friend Bob Schuller, "Life is like an echo. What you give out is what comes back." The mood you give out to people is what comes back to you. The Bible says, ". . . Whatsoever a man soweth, that shall he also reap" (Galatians 6:7 KJV).

3. REFUSE TO SURRENDER THE LEADERSHIP OF YOUR LIFE TO BAD MOODS.   Unfortunately, many people allow their moods to run their lives. When they feel good, you can count on them to do what they said they would, but if they

are in a down mood swing, they drop off like dead flies. Everyone has a bad mood sometime, but we don't have to give in to our bad moods. One thing about catering to a bad mood is that the more you give in to it, the more it takes over the control of your life. Whatever you do, don't surrender the leadership of your life to bad moods.

How many times we've expressed the words, "I don't feel like it," as if a low mood excuses us from following through on our commitments and responsibilities. Do you know that the best things in life have been accomplished by people who, a lot of the time, didn't feel like it, but went ahead and did it anyway?

Tom Dempsey is the kind of person who did it anyway. Tom was born without half a foot and only a stub of a right arm. But he didn't let that stop him. As a boy he wanted to play sports like the other boys. He had a burning desire to play football.

Because of his determination, his parents had an artificial foot made for him. It was made of wood. The wooden foot was encased in a specially designed football shoe. Hour after hour, day after day, whether or not Tom felt like it, he would practice kicking the football with his wooden foot. He would push himself to make field goals at greater and greater distances.

The payoff came when a few years ago he kicked a record-breaking sixty-three-yard field goal as a professional kicker to give his team, the Saints, a winning score of nineteen to seven over the Detroit Lions. Nearly 67,000 football fans, who were present to witness this achievement, screamed and yelled in appreciation for Tom Dempsey.

Tom Dempsey is a champion because he refused to surrender the leadership of his life to the negative.

The Bible gives the word that we need to hear and apply in our lives. "... Be ye stedfast, unmoveable, always abounding in the work of the Lord ..." (1 Corinthians 15:58 KJV).

4. UNLOAD YOUR BURDENS UPON THE LORD.   When the burdens of life are weighing you down, take them to the Lord in prayer. The Scriptures tell us, "Cast your burdens upon the Lord" (*see* Psalms 55:22). Why should we be all burdened down when we can take whatever it is that is bothering us to the Lord in prayer and let go of it and let God have it?

The story is told of an expedition of scientists who went on a mission to capture a particular specimen of monkeys in the jungle of Africa. It was essential that the monkeys be brought back alive and unharmed.

Using their knowledge of monkeys' ways, the scientists devised a trap consisting of a small jar with a long, narrow neck. Inside the jar was placed a handful of nuts.

A number of the jars were prepared and staked out, while the scientists calmly waited close by, confident they would make their catch. Sure enough, the monkeys came and thrust their paws into the long neck to take a fistful of nuts. But when they tried to withdraw the prize, they could not get their clenched fists through the small opening at the top. Unwilling to release the fist and let go of the nuts, the monkeys all remained caught in the bottles. When the scientists returned, they easily took the monkeys captive.

We smile at the monkeys, thinking how foolish they are.

But how many times we get all bound up and down in our spirits simply because we are clinging to things we should let go of?

The songwriter said it this way:

> O WHAT PEACE WE OFTEN FORFEIT,
> O WHAT NEEDLESS PAIN WE BEAR,
> ALL BECAUSE WE DO NOT CARRY
> EV'RYTHING TO GOD IN PRAYER.
>
> JOSEPH SCRIVEN

5. IN EVERYTHING GIVE THANKS. A big step to take that will help lift you out of a bad mood is to discover and practice the thanks principle. What is the thanks principle? It is found in 1 Thessalonians 5:18 (KJV), "In every thing give thanks: for this is the will of God in Christ Jesus concerning you." If you will do this, it will give your moods a positive lift.

Wilson Cline apparently was a very successful businessman. Yet he suffered from periods of deep depression. Wilson had been to some of the finest doctors in our city and to one of our best known psychiatrists. Yet he still found no relief from his deep depression.

I asked Wilson if he was willing to try a spiritual experiment. He confessed at this point that he was willing to do anything that would get him up out of his downer. I turned to this verse, we read it together and I said, "Now this week I want you, the first thing in the morning when you get up, to give thanks to God for something. Throughout the day I want you to keep on thanking God for everything that comes to your mind. Whatever happens during your day, just keep thanking God."

I cautioned Wilson that this was really going to feel strange at first, but to do it anyway and to keep on doing it. I got him to agree that he would try this spiritual exercise for one week.

At the end of that first week the change in Wilson was fantastic. Overflowing with excitement, he related how about the third day into the exercise, his spirit began to lift until now he was experiencing a continual flow of the joy of the Lord. Practicing the principle of thanksgiving on a consistent daily basis had opened the door to a flow of joy in his life.

I DARE YOU TO—
IN EVERYTHING GIVE THANKS.

You will notice that this thanks verse does not say, "For everything give thanks," but, "In every thing give thanks." Not everything that comes into our life is good in itself.

I confess to you that I didn't enjoy the inconvenience I was caused the other day when my car wouldn't start. I will also tell you that it doesn't make me overflow with joy to see some of the suffering I've seen in the lives of people for whom I care deeply. But in the midst of these reverses, I thank God that He is still in charge, that He's in control. I thank Him because He is Lord of all and over all. Yes: "In every thing give thanks."

As you dare to practice this thanks principle, you are going to discover the truth of Romans 8:28 (KJV): "And we know that all things work together for good to them that love God. . . ." Thank God that He is at work bringing good out of bad. He has a miraculous way of putting it all together so the final outcome is for our good.

6. TURN YOUR DIAL ON THE POSITIVE. Your mind may be likened to a radio receiver. Your decision maker is the tuner dial. You can tune in to any frequency you choose to. The other morning when I was driving to work, about halfway to the office I suddenly realized that I was irritated, and then it dawned on me that the station I was tuned to was playing music that was anything but calming and soothing. Immediately I turned the station over to my favorite station that always has what I call good music. Sure enough there was soft, quiet, soothing, uplifting music. And when I got the right station tuned in, my mood was lifted.

All around you there are negative things, and there are positive things. Somewhere right in the middle of your mind, you have a tuning dial, and you choose whether to tune in the negative or the positive. If you tune in the negative, you are going to find yourself cast down. On the other hand, if you tune in the positive to see the good, the lovely and dwell on what's right, you are going to be lifted in your spirit. The Scripture says, "As a man thinketh in his heart so is he" (*see* Proverbs 23:7).

To give yourself a positive lift:

- Center on what you have, not what you don't have
- Center on what you can do, not on what you can't do
- Center on what is right in your life, not on what is wrong
- Center on what you can do for others, not what you wish they would do for you

7. How Do You Get Up When You're Down? By Planting a Positive Seed! A couple of years ago I received a letter from a mother of a retarded child. Marie shared how she had cried for days and nights over her retarded child. Sometimes she cried for a child whom she knew could never be normal. Most of the time she cried for herself and the unbearable hardship she faced.

Marie William told me that she never got on top of her situation until she did two things. First of all, she began to practice the verse "In every thing give thanks," and then she began to pray that prayer every morning first thing. "Thank You God, for my retarded child. Thank You that You're going to help him to become the best person he could be. Thank You God, because You're going to help me to grow as a person through having a retarded son."

The second thing Marie practiced as a way to get her out of a negative cycle and bring her into a positive flow of life. She planted a positive seed. The thing she saw was that she wasn't very happy. Instead of feeling sorry for herself, she needed to do what she could to make others happy. What could she do? God dropped a beautiful idea into her mind.

The special school for retarded children needed volunteers. She gave of herself by volunteering to help the school every afternoon. By working with other children and trying to make them happy, she came to understand better her own child and his handicap and what she could do to help him. Yes, she was worn out by the time night came. But, one night when she was reflecting back over the weeks, it dawned on her that she had found a new joy.

GIVE YOURSELF AWAY,
AND YOU WILL FIND YOURSELF.
PLANT A POSITIVE SEED,
AND GOD WILL USE IT TO GIVE A MIRACLE.
MAKE OTHERS HAPPIER, AND YOU WILL FIND
YOUR HAPPINESS.

8. LIFT YOUR VOICE TO GOD IN PRAISE. I have saved the most exhilarating point to last. What I am going to share with you now is a step beyond the principle of thanksgiving. It is the greatest emotional lift that there is. What is it? *It is the principle of praise.* The Scriptures tell us to do what is good for our moods when it says, "Rejoice in the Lord always: and again I say, Rejoice" (Philippians 4:4 KJV).

BE DELIGHTED IN THE LORD.

Biweekly on Thursday nights we tape our New Hope television programs. It has been our practice to start taping promptly at 5:30 and to continue until we've finished, whatever the hour. Television is a magnificent opportunity to reach people where they are and be used of God to heal their hurts and build their dreams. Being the speaker on our program, it is essential that I be well prepared and at my best for every taping. In order to do this, I make it a practice to block out my other responsibilities on the scheduled taping day and concentrate solely on what God wants to do with my life through television.

In spite of well-planned good intentions, on one of the recent taping days I had some really large problems connected with our building project for our church, which demanded my immediate attention. After wrestling with these weighty problems all day, I went to the evening television taping flat out of energy.

While I made it through the first program taping all right, by the time for the second program taping I was so tired that my knees were weak and my mind was fuzzy. At my point of need the Holy Spirit brought the lifting praise principle to remembrance in my mind.

I left the studio and walked off into an isolated area where I could be alone with God, lifted my voice, and praised the Lord. As I praised the Lord from the inside out, suddenly it was as if He reached down and lifted me up right to where I needed to be—on the heights with Him. I went back in to speak with fresh newness and most of all, the anointing of God's Spirit upon me.

Hallelujah! Yes, Praise the Lord! Praise him in his Temple, and in the heavens he made with mighty power. Praise him for his mighty works. Praise his unequaled greatness. Praise him with the trumpet and with lute and harp. Praise him with the tambourines and processional. Praise him with stringed instruments and horns. Praise him with the cymbals, yes, loud clanging cymbals. Let everything alive give praises to the Lord! *You* praise him! Hallelujah!

Psalms 150 TLB

LET'S JUST PRAISE THE LORD!

Self-evaluation

Chart your own mood patterns on a daily basis for one month.

10 Ecstatic
9 Elated
8 Excited
7 Happy
6 Good feelings
5 Neutral
4 Unpleasant feelings
3 Sad
2 Self-pity
1 Depressed

Each day select the number by the word that best represents your overall mood for the day and place the correct dot in the day you are on. Track your own mood swing each day by connecting the dots.

Help With Your Habits

Every night for years Thomas Buchanan, the lighthouse keeper, went to sleep to the restless, unceasing, lonely sound of the bell on the buoy near the lighthouse. It has been reported that he was never conscious of the ceaseless tolling of the bell as it rolled and rocked with the motions of the sea, until one night, suddenly the bell stopped its ringing. Immediately the lighthouse keeper sat straight up in bed, startled, and said to his wife, "What was that?"

I think that we find this story amusing because it has an element of truth that hits home in each of our lives. You see, we are all creatures of habit much more than we realize. In my own life every morning I get up about the same time, brush my teeth, shave, put on my jogging clothes, do the same calisthenics. Then I jog three miles down the same path in automatic gear while my mind talks to the Lord and receives and thinks on exciting ideas. When I return home, I shower, eat my breakfast, get in the car and drive the exact same road to the office every morning. My trip to the office is such a habit that on those exceptional mornings when I am supposed to be going in another direction, if I don't really consciously think about it, I find myself automatically going down the same road that leads to my office.

I am not the only creature of habit; I'd venture to say that you are, too. Would you please allow me to illustrate this to you? Right now, fold your arms. It's easy to fold your arms, you've done it hundreds of times. Are your arms folded?

With your arms folded I want you to notice which arm you have on top of the other. Is it the right one or the left one? Here comes the second step in this fun experiment. Ready? Quickly reverse the way your arms are folded. Hard to do, isn't it? Why? Because we are in the habit of folding our arms the same without thinking. To reverse the way we fold our arms takes the effort of thinking about it and acting upon that thought.

A large portion of your life is automatically run by your habits. It has been estimated by experts that 80 percent of everything we do from the time we get up until we go to bed is out of habit.

Habits conserve for us what we have learned yesterday. A habit helps us to repeat the behavior automatically without having to think or to learn all over again. What a wonderful servant a habit can be!

Without the help of habits, all of our lives would be much more complicated. Do you realize that if it were not for habit, you could not open your front door and take a walk outside without stopping to think about how to take each step?

Do you remember when you were first learning to drive, how it took tedious concentration to make those constant steering adjustments right and left as you drove your car? But as you practiced, your driving became more automatic, until finally you developed the habit of making those same adjustments without even thinking about it. Habits save us energy and effort.

What is a habit? A habit is a wonderful invention that God has placed within each of us. You might say it is like a built-in automatic pilot. A habit is a thought or action that we have repeated until it has become automatic, and we do it without stopping to decide.

There are good habits, and there are bad habits. Habits can:

- Be your friend or be your enemy
- Help you or hurt you
- Serve you or enslave you
- Work for you or work against you
- Aid you in your Christian witness or damage your Christian witness

GOD CREATED AND SAVED YOU TO BE THE MASTER OF GOOD HABITS, INSTEAD OF THE SLAVE TO BAD HABITS

Unfortunately, in our society, the word *habit* has gotten a bad name. We have made a word with unlimited positive potential into a very negative word. In most of the writings today, what we read about is the drinking habit, the drug habit, the smoking habit, overeating habit, swearing habit, and the illicit-sex habit.

The exciting news is that you can choose and develop habits that, rather than working against you, can work for you. One of the beautiful results of being Christ's disciple is to "... be a new and different person, holy and good ..." (Ephesians 4:24 TLB). This begins by "becoming a brand new person inside" (*see* 2 Corinthians 5:17), at which time a new life is begun. The moment we receive Jesus as Lord into our lives He gives us the beautiful name *Christian.* Then as we follow Him, putting off old defeating habits and putting on new, positive, life-building habits, we grow into the name *Christian,* so that being truly a Christian means ridding oneself of bad habits and selecting and building into one's life good habits. It's true that old habits do not die easily, while good habits do not come alive without effort and determination. But I believe, with Christ's help, you can do it. You can eliminate habits that work against you, and you can build positive habits that will work for you, to give you more and more of the good life in your daily living.

Understand How Habits Are Formed

Before we can eliminate bad habits in our lives and establish good ones, it is necessary for us to understand how habits are formed. *Every habit you and I have has been learned.* Now, if a certain habit has been learned, it can also be unlearned. There is no habit that cannot be dropped from or added to your repertory. Good news: you can, with Christ's help, change for the better.

First, let us see that some habits are learned in response to given stimuli. For example, if a child gets what he wants by screaming, he soon learns to scream to get what he wants. Thus he grows up with the habit of screaming to get his own way. This is why, as parents, we must be on guard not to reward our children for misbehavior. On the other hand, by complimenting or rewarding good behavior, we can reinforce a habit of good behavior in our children.

The second way that habits are formed is by imitation. We all tend to do what our heroes or role models do. Millions of kids have been turned on to drugs by imitating one of the rock stars who openly advocates drugs as the way to go. This is why it is so important that our children and young people have the right heroes to follow and imitate.

Children are great imitators. When my youngest son, Scott, was not quite two years of age, he liked to follow me into the bathroom. Guess what he insisted on doing? He had a little red toothbrush, and every morning while I brushed my teeth, he had to brush his teeth—all of them! Think of it, at nineteen months, he was forming a good habit of brushing his teeth every morning. How was he learning this habit? By imitation. Parents, older brother and sister, take warning. A little boy or a little girl is following in your steps. The habits that they are learning from you they will be living with for a lifetime.

The third way habits develop is through repetition. Do something once, and it is easier to do it the second time. You do it the third, fourth, fifth time, and before long you have the habit. Someone has said, "A rope woven with threads of twine soon forms a rope too thick to be broken." Understand this and use it to build good habits into your daily life.

The less painful way to cure a bad habit is never to get started in it. An ounce of prevention is worth a pound of cure. Take the health destructive habit of smoking, which is offensive to a lot of non-smokers. How does anyone ever get started smoking? By smoking one cigarette, then another, and another, and almost before he knows it, he has a habit. It has been estimated that 95 percent of all smokers in America acquired the habit before their twenty-second birthday. The majority of these people wish they had never gotten started. What does this teach us? Not to start anything that we do not want to become a habit. A word of wisdom to all of us is, before you start something, take the long look and ask yourself, "If this is to become a habit in my life, will it have a good lasting result or a bad one?" The wise person chooses and cultivates good habits, while rejecting actions that, repeated, will lead to the enslavement to bad habits.

Use repetition to learn good habits. When our children were younger, Margi and I learned to solve the problem of being at each other's throats by the time we got to church by choosing and cultivating a good habit of working together. Previously, I had been used to running off to the church and leaving her at home to care for and prepare the small children for church. I made a decision that I would do everything I could to help to make the Sunday-morning preparation harmonious, instead of a disaster.

We made it a habit together to pitch in, bathe the children on Saturday night, lay out their clothes, and do whatever we could to prepare ahead of time. Then on Sunday morning we both pitched in, helping dress the children, prepare their breakfast, comb their hair, working together to do whatever needed to be done, so that we could leave the house in a spirit of love and preparation by 8:00.

What a difference choosing and cultivating these good habits in preparation for going to church made in our family life. Instead of everyone being uptight from hurrying, scurrying, and rushing, we found ourselves ready on time, prepared and relaxed. Besides that, we all had fun working together to achieve this. It became a good habit that worked not only for individual good, but for the good of our whole family.

SOW AN ACT AND YOU REAP A HABIT.
SOW A HABIT AND YOU REAP A CHARACTER.
SOW A CHARACTER AND YOU REAP A DESTINY.

Put Good Habits to Work for You

There are infinite possibilities when it comes to good habits that you can form at your will. With each good habit you form comes an aid to better living for you and yours. Take a sheet of paper right now and write down every good habit that you wish was yours. In order to get your creative juices going, read through the following list of good habits:

Smiling is a good habit
Being attentive to your wife or husband is a good habit
Attending church is a good habit
Being cheerful to your loved ones in the morning is a good habit
Daily exercise is a good habit
Limiting the amount you eat is a good habit
Making your bed the first thing in the morning is a good habit
Being prompt is a good habit
Being honest is a good habit
Eating a well-balanced, nutritious breakfast is a good habit
Saving money is a good habit
Paying your bills on time is a good habit
Listening is a good habit
Being courteous to salespeople and service-station attendants is a good habit
Keeping your clothes clean and pressed is a good habit
Being positive and optimistic is a good habit

Spending a quiet time with God each day is a tremendous
   habit

Admittedly a good habit will not begin in your life by
mere wishful thinking. It's not going to happen just because
you think it might be a good idea. If this desired action is
going to become a repeated part of your life, then it's going
to take a decision, a commitment, and repeated effort on
your part to make this good habit a reality.

Enriching habits can be yours. You can have them, if you
will put forth the concentrated effort. A little concentrated
effort now will bring you tremendous yield in the days
ahead. Every good habit that you consciously acquire will
serve to enrich your life manyfold.

Stop Allowing Self-defeating Habits to Be Your Master

You were created by God to be the master of your habits,
not a slave to destructive habits. You have been chosen by
the Lord Jesus Christ and empowered by His Spirit within
to become the victor over any and all destructive habits that
drag you down.

What is a bad habit? A bad habit is any attitude or action
that holds you back and keeps you from being at your best.
A bad habit is a behavior that harms you or another person.
A bad habit is anything that separates you from God. A bad
habit is any action or attitude that mars your Christian witness.

Bad habits are not only smoking, drunkenness, overeating, and being unfaithful to one's mate. Although not as
well advertised as other sinful habits, the habit of negative

thinking can be just as destructive as bad behavior habits.

From a very early age Diana showed a great deal of natural talent and potential to become an outstanding concert pianist. But unfortunately, she had a mother who had a bad habit of harsh criticism that she leveled repeatedly at her daughter's playing. Unfortunately for Diana, she picked up the same bad habit of negative thinking and applied it to herself, thinking that she was never good enough.

As a young pianist Diana performed brilliantly at the piano keyboard, but if she made one small mistake, first her mother would scold her without mercy, then she, herself, would continue the berating. All the while she was doing well she thought she was incompetent. This habit of negative nitpicking completely wiped out Diana's competence. Now in her mid-twenties, when she has the ability and developed natural gifts to be a brilliant concert pianist, she refuses to play in front of anyone. As faulty as her negative thinking is, it has become an automatic habit that is literally wiping her out.

With Christ's help I believe that, if you would choose to, you can wipe out both bad behavioral habits and bad thinking habits. And as you do you are going to become so much more a positive, free, happy person.

How to Become Free From the Habit that Binds You

1. ADMIT YOUR OWN BAD HABIT OR HABITS.   Be honest with yourself. Others can see your bad habit; why can't you? Who are you kidding, anyway? I dare you to test any doubtful habit in your life with these two questions: *Does it hurt me? Does it hinder me?* If the answer is yes, then you

need to come to grips with the fact that you are being mastered by a bad habit.

2. BEFORE YOU CAN MASTER A BAD HABIT, YOU MUST MAKE UP YOUR MIND THAT YOU ARE GOING TO BECOME A QUITTER.   Let's face it, no bad habit is going to vanish by itself. Ordinarily I tell people never to quit. But when it comes to bad habits, the only way to be a winner is to become a quitter.

Talk to God until you believe with His help you can do it. "I can do all things through Christ which strengtheneth me" (Philippians 4:13 KJV). With Jesus as your Master you can together master this bad habit.

3. DON'T WASTE YOUR ENERGY CONDEMNING YOURSELF.   Jesus said, "Neither do I condemn thee: go, and sin no more" (John 8:11 KJV). Far better to spend your energy in constructive changing than in self-condemnation. You make mistakes—mistakes don't make you. View the times you have tried and not made it as just warm-ups for the final battle to victory. If you commit yourself to becoming master over this habit, you can be confident that Christ is going to help you win the battle.

4. SET A TIME AND GET STARTED.   You will never be rid of that habit until you take the initiative and set the date to begin. I suggest you mark your planned beginning date in bold ink on your calendar.

Watch out for the common enemy: procrastination. Anything we put off until tomorrow usually never gets done. What makes you think tomorrow will make it any easier to do? You know inside that the sooner you get started the better. So why not do it now? *Now* spelled backwards is *won*. Get started now and you will take one giant step to becoming a winner over that defeating habit.

5. VISUALIZE YOURSELF WINNING. Researchers have dramatized the impact of visualization for us by finding that 80 percent of all buying decisions are made as a result of visualization. The ability that God has given us to picture it in our minds before it becomes reality is a tremendous tool. Today's dreams become tomorrow's realities.

Make use of visualization to help you change your habit. As much as I like to eat desserts, I have found that I can resist any fatty treat by simply picturing maggots crawling around all over the goody. This picture will curb my appetite every time.

Change the picture in your mind from negative to positive. Instead of seeing yourself as fat, picture yourself as the way you really want to be—slim and trim. See yourself as responding positively to new ideas. Picture yourself as a winner over that habit that has so long bound you. Fix your mind on that picture of the new you, and it will act like a magnet, pulling you upward to achievement.

6. EXPECT SOME TEMPORARY PAIN. Understand that you are going to experience some mental, physical anguish in withdrawing from this habit. But remember, the pain is only temporary. Look at the continuing pain this habit will bring into your life if you persist in it. It is much better to suffer temporary pain than to go on and on suffering the consequences of a bad habit. For example, being overweight could very well result in your premature death. Deny the lesser to gain the greater. There is no gain over bad habits

without a little temporary pain. And the victory that you are going to gain is certainly worth that temporary discomfort.

The joy and excitement of having shed those pounds, given up the weed, gotten off the booze, is well worth the effort. Listen to the flowing, exciting testimonies of others who have gained the victory over bad habits. Aren't they happy? I tell you it is going to do something for your self-respect, too. It is going to make you feel so good about yourself.

7. NEVER GIVE UP UNTIL YOU HAVE WON THE VICTORY. Whatever you do, don't ever give up. With Christ's help, victory over the habit is yours if you will keep putting forth the effort, more effort, and never give up. Deny the lesser, and you will gain the greater.

REPLACE ONE BAD HABIT WITH A GOOD ONE.

Harold Smith had a bad habit that was harmful not only to him but all the members of his family. The moment he opened the door in returning from a day's work, he would come in and start yelling at his wife because dinner wasn't ready. All the time she was trying her best, but with four small children, two of them still in diapers, she had her hands full. By the time Harold came home she was ready to collapse into his arms, but what she got instead of help was being yelled at by a man who was thinking about no one but himself.

In the midst of some very fine Christian counseling, the counselor was able to confront Harold about this bad destructive habit. For the first time, Harold saw how selfish he was being and what his habit of yelling at everyone was doing to his wife and children and how it was making everyone miserable.

In the conversation with the counselor, it came out that Harold's yelling habit would create deep resentments inside his wife. When they would go to bed and he would want her response sexually, she would be turned off.

In a learning conversation with the counselor, Harold made up his mind that he was going to put a stop to this bad habit of yelling the moment he came in the door. He took the suggestion of the counselor that he replace the bad habit with some positive action. The positive action was that he take the children, go down to the family room, and spend some time with them while his wife finished getting the dinner.

This took a lot of effort on Harold's part. For the first couple of nights of working at changing his habits he felt strangely awkward not yelling his head off and even more by sitting down calmly and looking after the children. But he was a fast learner, and after a couple of weeks, he had a new habit mastered that made him feel better about himself.

The payoff was that, by replacing a bad habit with a good habit, his children were responding to him as a father whom they loved. His wife became responsive in the bedroom, and there was a whole new kind of understanding and love reigning in the home.

WITH CHRIST'S HELP,
MASTER YOUR HABITS
AND ENJOY A RICHER, MORE MEANINGFUL LIFE.

Self-evaluation

1. List all bad habits that you would like to do away with.

2. List the bad habit that you would like to change first. Set the date when you plan to get started.

3. Is there a good habit that you might replace this bad one with?
   If the answer is yes, then write down the good habit that you want to replace the bad one with.

4. Write down all the good habits that you would like to choose and make a part of your life.

5. Write down the two good habits that you most desire to make a part of your daily life.

6. Set time and date when you plan to get started on making these two good habits a part of your life.

8

Fourteen Principles to Gain Financial Freedom

WHILE CONDUCTING a money seminar, I began by asking this question: "Why is it so difficult to manage money?" These are some of the answers that I received: inflation, easy credit, pressure to keep up with the Joneses, the power of advertisement, high interest rates, not making enough money, trying to give children too much, unable to say no to salesmen, and many other similar answers.

Finally one lady hit the nail right on the head when she said, "I believe it's difficult to manage money because it is hard work, and being a little on the lazy side, we avoid hard work." It is true that there is no other area of life that requires more determination and self-discipline to manage than the area of money.

Five Financial Realities That We Do Not Like to Face

1. YOUR MONEY IS NOT GOING TO MANAGE ITSELF.   Fail to manage your money, and you have sown the seeds of financial failure. The number-one pitfall that people fall into is to think that somehow by some magic their money is going to manage itself. Nothing could be further from the truth. The plain truth is, if you don't manage your money, no one will.

2. OF FAR MORE CONSEQUENCE THAN HOW MUCH MONEY YOU MAKE IS WHAT YOU ARE DOING WITH WHAT YOU ARE NOW EARNING. Researchers tell us that often, the more money that people make, the poorer money managers they become. You say, "What? How could this be?" It's because they live under the false illusion that making more and more money will solve their money problems. Unless a person manages his money, the more money he makes, the more money problems he is going to have. I knew a man who made an average income and had some money problems, but as a result of successfully marketing a new gadget he had invented, his income was multiplied ten times within a year. At the end of that year, instead of having ten times the money problems, it appeared to me that he had a hundred times the problems. The year that he made $80,000, he actually had to file for bankruptcy. How you manage what you earn is far more important than how much you earn.

3. A PERSON CANNOT AFFORD TO SPEND MORE THAN HE MAKES. A sixth grader could tell you that if you make $200 a week and spend $212 a week, it is not going to be very long until you are in financial trouble. Reality—you cannot afford to spend more money than you make.

4. EASY CREDIT ON ITEMS THAT DEPRECIATE RAPIDLY IS A BUMMER. The item is used, worn-out, gone, and what do you have left? A bill and more debt. Question—if you cannot afford to pay cash for it now, how can you afford to pay it later, plus 18 percent compounded interest?

5. NO MATTER HOW MUCH YOU MAKE, THERE ARE MANY THINGS YOU CANNOT AFFORD. This is one difficult reality that is hard for us, who have been brought up in an affluent

society, to accept. I for one like to think that I can say yes to anything I want for any member of my family wants. But the stark financial reality is that there are many things I cannot afford to buy. Let's face it, we are all in the same boat. There are a lot of things that none of us can afford to buy. So why not accept financial reality and say no. We need to say no.

The Challenge of Money Management

Did you know that God trusts you? That's right! The One who owns it all keeps placing some of it in your care to manage. In Matthew 25, Jesus tells the parable of the talents. The story illustrates how God gives to each of us different portions to manage. According to Jesus' explanation, it is not the amount we are given that is most important, but how well we manage what is placed under our supervision. It is both a sobering and a challenging truth that each of us is accountable to God the Father for how we manage our money.

To fail to manage what God places in our care is to be the same as an unfaithful servant. To squander it away is to be unfaithful to the truth that He places in our care. On the other hand, to do a good job in managing what He gives us is to earn the right to handle more. To all those who do a good job God gives the abundant increase.

CAN GOD TRUST YOU WITH MONEY?

I know that you want to do a good job managing your money. You want to know how you can excel in money management? Here is how. Practice this absolute principle: deny the lesser to gain the greater.

Principles to Gain Financial Freedom

1. GIVE 10 PERCENT TO GOD—OFF THE TOP!   The Bible calls this tithing. It happens to be a most important first step, not only in finding the solution to your money problems, but also in becoming successful in the handling of all that God has given you, plus the increase He is going to bring to you as you put Him first.

To get God's best you have to give Him your best. Don't kid yourself—you can't give God leftovers and fool Him into thinking you are giving Him your best. There is no bigger fool than he who keeps fooling himself. You do want God's very best and highest in life, don't you? Then follow the teaching of Scripture found in Proverbs 3:6, 9 (TLB):

> In everything you do, put God first, and he will direct you and crown your efforts with success. . . . Honor the Lord by giving him the first part of all your income, and he will fill your barns with wheat and barley and overflow your wine vats with the finest wines.

It has been my observation from working with hundreds of people that those who never learn to practice the principle of tithing are forever having multiple money problems. On the other hand, tithing alone does not guarantee financial success, but it is the most important beginning step to take in managing your money. And as you tithe you can count not only on God's help in your financial life but also on His bountiful blessings.

2. WORK HARD.   As someone has said, "There is no sub-
stitute for hard work, and there is no success for laziness."
The Bible says it this way, "Lazy men are soon poor; hard
workers get rich" (Proverbs 10:4 TLB). If you want the best
things in life, then you have to deny your natural laziness
and develop the good habit of putting yourself wholeheart-
edly into work.

3. SEIZE THE OPPORTUNITY TO BETTER YOURSELF.   The
Bible says, "A wise youth makes hay while the sun shines,
but what a shame to see a lad who sleeps away his hour of
opportunity" (Proverbs 10:5 TLB). Be alert! Opportunities to
advance are coming.

4. SEEK AS MUCH COUNSEL AND ADVICE AS YOU CAN GET.
Before making any major financial decision like buying a
house, going into business, or making a sizeable investment,
seek out the counsel of godly people. "A fool thinks he
needs no advice, but a wise man listens to others." (Proverbs
12:15 TLB). You will be amazed at how many fine experts are
willing to give you good, sound advice free of charge, if you
will only ask.

The person who seeks out all of the expert financial advice he can get before making a decision is miles ahead.
Usually when we avoid the counsel of Christian advisers it is
because inside we know there is something wrong with what
we want to do. Proverbs tells us, "Plans go wrong with too
few counselors; many counselors bring success" (Proverbs
15:22 TLB). Be wise and accept the fact that many counselors
are better than one.

5. DON'T BE TOO PROUD TO ADMIT YOU'VE MADE A FINAN-
CIAL MISTAKE.   Sometime or other, everyone makes a fi-

nancial mistake. The sooner one admits his mistake, takes his lumps, and gets out of it, the wiser he is. How foolish it is to be too proud to admit your mistake and keep getting in deeper and deeper. The Scripture warns us, "Pride goes before destruction and haughtiness before a fall" (Proverbs 16:18 TLB).

6. DON'T COSIGN ANOTHER PERSON'S NOTES.   "It is poor judgment to countersign another's note, to become responsible for his debts" (Proverbs 17:18 TLB).

7. BEFORE MAKING A FINANCIAL DECISION, GATHER ALL THE POSSIBLE FACTS.   There are many people who will not tell an out-and-out lie to you, but on the other hand, will not tell you all the facts unless you ask. Assume nothing until you have checked it out for certain. A friend of mine recently had a terrific expense of having to exterminate termites in the home he had purchased. A close check of the foundation before closing the deal could have saved him a lot of money. The Bible says, "What a shame—yes, how stupid!—to decide before knowing the facts!" (Proverbs 18:13 TLB).

8. IF YOUR PRICE IS FAIR, STICK TO IT.   Proverbs 20:14 (TLB) gives us this appropriate advice concerning someone trying to beat down your fair price. " 'Utterly worthless!' says the buyer as he haggles over the price. But afterwards he brags about his bargain!"

9. BE HONEST IN ALL YOUR DEALINGS.   It's true, financial gain can be gained by cheating. But sooner or later the temporary gain turns grimy. The Bible says, "A fortune can be

made from cheating, but there is a curse that goes with it" Proverbs 20:21 TLB).

10. BE CAREFUL ABOUT SPECULATION.   Wise persons heed this verse, "Steady plodding brings prosperity; hasty speculation brings poverty." (Proverbs 21:5 TLB).

11. LIVE DEBT FREE.   To be free as God intended for you to live, it is necessary for you to avoid the debt trap. And if you are in the debt trap, then take whatever radical steps are necessary to get out of depressing debt as quickly as possible. Borrowing for a house or a car is one thing, but being enslaved to charge accounts and easy credit is a downer. Depressing debt robs us of the freedoms that God intended for us to enjoy. As Proverbs 22:7 (TLB) says, "Just as the rich rule the poor, so the borrower is servant to the lender."

12. BUILD YOUR BUSINESS FIRST, BEFORE YOU BUILD YOUR HOUSE.   This wise truth is laid down in Proverbs 24:27 (TLB): "Develop your business first before building your house." If you make your business strong and healthy, you will have more than enough money to pay for a nice home.

13. PREPARE FOR FINANCIAL NEEDS AHEAD BY SAVING NOW.   If you own a car, if you own a house, if you have children, if you own anything mechanical, and if you are alive, sooner or later you are going to have an unexpected financial emergency. Someone is going to get sick, the car is going to stop running and need repair, or as happened to us this week, your furnace may go out. To those who have saved and prepared ahead of time, a financial emergency is just another happening in life. To the person who has not saved, a financial emergency is always a major calamity. "A

sensible man watches for problems ahead and prepares to meet them. The simpleton never looks, and suffers the consequences" (Proverbs 27:12 TLB).

14. AVOID GET-RICH-QUICK SCHEMES. When someone promises you a lot of money for nothing, you had better beware. "Trying to get rich quick is evil and leads to poverty" (Proverbs 28:22 TLB).

DENY THE LESSER
AND
GAIN BY MANAGING YOUR MONEY.

Self-evaluation

1. Make a list of persons and situations in your life toward which you have negative feelings. Beside each one write down what positive action you need to take to change your thinking from negative to positive.

a. _____

_____

_____

b. _____

_____

_____

c. _____

_____

_____

d. _____

_____

_____

2. Make a list of every positive thing you can think of in
   your life._____

   _____

   _____

   _____

   _____

   _____

   _____

   _____

   _____

   _____

   _____

Six Ways to Keep Positive in a Negative World

How do you keep positive when negative things keep happening in your life? How do you keep positive when everyone else around you is being negative? Let's admit it, it's not easy to keep positive in a world in which the large majority of people are negative.

We live in a very negative world. In case you don't think so, I challenge you to pick up today's newspaper and evaluate it line for line. If the paper is like the average daily newspaper, after you have judged each article on the criterion of whether it is positive or negative and calculated the results, you will discover that 90 percent or more of what you have read is not positive but negative. What some news reporters do is pull out the negative and blow it up until, after a while, that's all we see and hear. The abnormal is made out to be the normal. No wonder some people are coming to believe that no news is good news.

From my own experience in the past year and a half of being the leader in a huge building project for New Hope Community Church, being positive is not always easy. Our project has been caught in the midst of a recession. In talking to scores of bankers and financial leaders in our community I have discovered that they are not the most positive-thinking people in the world. Don't get me wrong—I like bankers, but from my own personal experience they look at things from the negative viewpoint. If I had allowed them to squeeze me into their negative mold of thinking, our inspiring project of building our dream church would not even have gotten off the ground, let alone become a reality.

Without PMA, which stands for Positive Mental Attitude, not one good thing can you achieve. Because without PMA, all you have is NMA which stands for Negative Mental Attitude. And with a negative mental attitude, a person does not even dare to start to do anything, no matter how worthwhile it is.

Some years ago two competing salesmen for shoe manufacturers arrived simultaneously in Africa to develop a market for their companies. Both men headed for the unexplored interior. After a few weeks, one of the salesmen cabled his company that he was returning home on the next boat because of the lack of sales opportunities. The natives did not wear shoes.

While the other salesman, who had PMA, sent off this telegram to his company: "Quick, send millions of pairs of shoes all sizes, colors, and styles, because the natives here have no shoes." The one man without a positive attitude saw nothing except the impossibilities, while the man with the positive attitude saw the opportunity and seized it. *What a difference our attitude makes.*

Which would you rather live with—PMA or NMA?
PMA—makes you feel good
NMA—can make you sick

PMA—can help you to see the best
NMA—can make you see the worst

PMA—lifts you
NMA—drags you down

PMA—makes you master over circumstances
NMA—makes you a slave of defeating circumstances

PMA—can win you friends and give you positive influence over others
NMA—can lose you friends and give you a negative influence over others

PMA—can make you more like Jesus
NMA—can make you more like the devil

Regardless of how anyone else chooses to think, if you really want a positive mental attitude, you can have it. How can you be positive in a negative world? Only one way: by using self-discipline not once, not twice, not three times, but again and again. To be positive in a negative world takes repeated self-discipline. And to keep positive, one must consciously, intentionally resist the negative and persist in choosing the positive.

You do not have to be squeezed into the mold of negative thinking that dominates so much of the world today. The Scriptures say it this way, "Don't let the world around you squeeze you into its own mould" (Romans 12:2 PHILLIPS). God has placed within you the power of choice to resist all of the negative influences and to fill your mind with the positive.

Six Ways to Keep Positive in a Negative World

1. Exercise Your Positive Choice!

I heard the other day about a man who had a day at the office where everything went wrong. First thing in the morning the bank called and told him that his business accounts were overdrawn. He had just hung up from that call, and his sales manager came in to tell him their biggest client was taking his business elsewhere.

While he was trying to work on these big problems, everybody else kept bothering him with their problems. At the close of this workday, feeling as if he'd been run over by a locomotive, he wasn't paying much attention to his driving, and he was stopped by a policeman and given a ticket. By the time he got home, he was in a terrible mood. When he sat down in his easy chair, all he wanted was peace and quiet.

His little boy, to his father's dismay, was rather unruly. He kept screaming, yelling, pestering him, demanding his attention. Finally the fed-up father shouted, "Get out of here and leave me alone."

Every day I meet people who are defeated by circumstances; they are overrun by what's happening to them; and they have given in to living with a negative mental attitude.

One of the great messages of Christianity is that no matter what happens in your life, you still have a choice. First of all, when God created you and made you, He gave you the marvelous power of choice. And second, in Christ's coming to be with us, we have the power available to be more than conquerors through Him that loved us and gave Himself for us. Jesus wants us to live with a victorious, overcoming power in our lives—to be victors, not helpless victims.

No matter what happens in your life, there is no such thing as a choiceless life. *You always have a choice!* You may face some very trying circumstances. You may face problems that seem unsolvable. Or in your home you may be having things happen that you feel are out of control. But, my friend, you still have a choice to make. Your choice between a positive mental attitude and a negative mental attitude will make all the difference in the conscious world you live in.

Years ago, Ella Wheeler Wilcox sat by the East River in New York, reflecting on the fact that persons coming from the very same home environment can turn out so differently. As she was sitting there, she saw some sailing vessels, pulling their way up the river to the docks and was inspired to write these powerful words:

> One ship drives east and another drives west
> With the self-same winds that blow.
> 'Tis the set of the sails
> And not the gales
> Which tells us the way to go.

In the midst of a tragic, terrible thing that happened in my life, I came across a story of Dr. Victor Frankl. As this courageous man stood under the glaring lights of the Gestapo court in a Nazi concentration camp soldiers took from him every earthly possession—his clothes, watch, even his wedding ring. Dr. Frankl said that as he stood there naked, his body shaved, publicly shamed, he was destitute but for one thing. It was something that no one could take away from him. He realized in that moment that he still had the power to choose his own attitude.

YOU ALWAYS HAVE A CHOICE.

No matter what is going on in your life, no matter how dark your situation may be, *you, and you alone, are the one who has the power to choose your own attitude.* What you choose to think, more than facts, more than circumstances, more than anything else, will determine the atmosphere in which you live. Choose to think the worst, and you will live in a gloomy world. Choose to look beyond the negative to see the positive, and a new world of beauty will open up before you. Beauty is all around you if you will look for it.

One Christmas, when our children were young, our neighbor put up his outdoor Christmas lights. As I drove in the driveway after a taxing day's work, I noticed the lights. *Wise guy,* I thought, *Margi's going to be after me now to put lights up on our house.* You see, choosing NMA was robbing me of enjoying the beauty of the lights.

Later on that evening, when I opened the front door, my three-year-old son, Scott, was standing by me and for the first time saw the lights across the street. He got so excited! He squealed, he jumped up and down, he was seeing for the first time the magic and the beauty of Christmas lights. Choosing a positive attitude, he was enjoying life.

Every day, in a hundred different situations, you and I

choose to either enjoy living with a positive mental attitude or drag through life with a negative mental attitude.

2. Fix Your Thoughts on What Is Good

The greatest book that was ever written on positive thinking is the Bible. In Philippians 4:8 we are given this nugget of truth: "Fix your thoughts on what is true and good and right. Think about things that are pure and lovely, and dwell on the fine, good things in others. Think about all you can praise God for and be glad about" (Philippians 4:8 TLB).

The word *fix* is an action word. It is something that you choose to do. The word *dwell* suggests to me that this is something that you need to keep on doing. The more you choose to fill your mind with positive thoughts, the more positive thinking will become a life-enriching habit.

Because of the intensity of the negative influence all around us, working overtime to squeeze us into a negative frame of mind, it is essential that we have daily times for renewing our thought life. Never have we needed to apply this verse to our lives more than in the present negative world in which we live. The Bible says, "And be not conformed to this world; but be transformed by the renewing of your minds, that you may prove what is good and acceptable, and the perfect will of God" (*see* Romans 12:2).

How do you renew your mind? By spending time reading and meditating on the Word of God and the things of God. Renewal comes as we fill our minds with power-packed verses like these:

> ... If you have faith as a grain of mustard seed, you shall say unto this mountain, remove hence to yonder

place; and it shall be removed: and nothing shall be impossible unto you.

See Matthew 17:20

For I am not ashamed of the gospel of Christ: for it is the power of God unto salvation to every one that believeth. . . .

Romans 1:16 KJV

I can do all things through Christ which strengthen-eth me.

Philippians 4:13 KJV

Choosing positive thoughts does not mean that you close your eyes to what is wrong. But it does mean that you keep whatever is wrong in total perspective of all that is right.

Clyde and Becky were a very happily married couple. Their love grew with the passing of each new year. When they were asked the secret of their marriage bliss, Clyde confessed that in the beginning years of their marriage they suffered from terrible open conflicts. In fact he said, "We even thought about calling it quits."

Then something happened that changed their lives. One day they decided to sit down and make a list of all the things they didn't like about each other. After they had finished their lists, they went through the painful experience of reading the long list of what they didn't like about each other out-loud. And as they courageously shared, they got it all out.

The next thing they did was to build a fire in the fireplace. Then they made a ceremony of burning up their lists of what was wrong with the other person. In that decisive moment, for the first time, just as they were, they accepted each other.

Then Clyde and Becky made another big decision to sit back down and each make a list of the other person's good points. After they had done this and shared out loud, they took the two positive lists into their bedroom, put them into an attractive picture frame, and proudly hung them on the wall.

From that life-changing day onward, through their many years of growing love, Clyde and Becky chose to keep centering on each other's good points instead of nit-picking at each other's faults. The self-discipline of fixing their thoughts on the good resulted in a happy marriage for this smart couple. The practice of this same principle will not only give your attitude a positive lift, but it will put a positive flow into all your relationships and will enrich your life.

3. Train Yourself to Be a Positive Reactionary

If you really want to live on top with a positive mental attitude, here is a fundamental principle that you must understand and put into practice:

NO MATTER WHAT HAPPENS
YOU CAN STILL CONTROL YOUR OWN REACTION.

There is an old Oriental saying, "You may not be able to keep the birds from flying over your head, but you can keep them from building a nest in your hair." How many times in our lives we react negatively to negative abuse and compound rather than solve our problems.

The other day my wife, Margi, made some delicious chocolate-chip cookies. For days I had been doing a good job of self-discipline in my eating, but chocolate-chip cookies seemed to be more temptation than I could overcome. As usual when she bakes chocolate-chip cookies, I quickly made a pig out of myself.

My wife told both our daughter, Ann, and our son, Scott, not to eat anymore, that they had had enough. She was afraid that eating anymore would make them sick. As I reached for another cookie in front of everyone she told me that I had had enough.

The truth was, that I had not only had enough, I had had too many. At that moment my rebellion raised its ugly head, and I wasn't about to let my wife dictate to me whether or not I could eat another cookie. So I showed her who was boss, and I ate the cookie.

You see, at the point of my negative rebellion, I lost my freedom to choose on a sensible basis whether or not I should eat another cookie. So instead of making a free choice, I just reacted to what she said and did the opposite.

You're laughing at me, but, how many times in the last week or so have you reacted negatively? I think one of the greatest challenges of life is to learn to react positively to negative happenings.

So big and so difficult is the challenge of learning to react positively to negative happenings, I know of no person alive who can accomplish this on a consistent daily basis without the help and power of the Lord Jesus Christ. Now I know there are people who, without claiming to be Christian, exercise their power of choice and think some pretty positive thoughts. But to be positive in spirit from the inside out when you are under attack is, from what I have observed, an impossibility without extraordinary God power within you. And Jesus Christ is the One who has come in supernatural power to live within us and through us.

JESUS CHRIST IS THE PERFECT EXAMPLE OF A POSITIVE REACTIONARY.

Into what kind of world did Jesus come to live and minister? It was a world in which two-thirds of the population were slaves. His own people, the Jewish race, lived under the forced rule and oppression of the corrupt Roman government. The hatred the Jewish people felt toward their oppressors was like a stopped-up pressure cooker building up steam, preparing to explode. Women were mistreated, and children were abused. Many suffered poverty and starvation. Yes, it was a very needy, disgruntled, negative world that Jesus lived in.

What did Jesus face? He faced the devil and all his crafty temptations. He faced the scorn and cynicism of the impossibility thinkers. Mockingly they sneered, "What good can come out of Nazareth?"

Throughout Jesus' public ministry, whenever He worked a miracle, there were those who refused to see the good in it. When Jesus made the crippled man to walk, all the nit-picking Pharisees could see was that He violated their man-made Sabbath laws.

There was a man out of his head, who lived among the tombs and acted like a madman. Jesus came to this tormented man and cast the demons out, giving him back his sanity. It was a miracle—the man was whole and at peace with himself. But all the negative businessmen of the community could see was that Jesus had cast the demons into their swine, which had run off the cliff. Seeing nothing except their loss, they begged Jesus to depart from their town.

Jesus touched a blind man who had been blind from birth and miraculously he received his sight. But all the negative critics wanted to know was, "Who sinned that this man was born blind?"

When Jesus died on the cross for our sins in the most positive act of love that has ever been shown, even those who were His closest disciples saw nothing but death. As Jesus paid it all, they lost hope. Talk about being negative—while the greatest event that has ever happened in history was taking place, they were totally defeated.

Why does man gravitate to the negative? Because of sin within him. How does one become positive? It must begin with an inner transformation by the power of the risen Jesus Christ. Jesus is not only our perfect example of a positive life, but He has come to put His positive life within us. Jesus said, "I am come that you might have life and you might have it more abundantly" (*see* John 10:10).

THROW OPEN THE DOOR OF YOUR LIFE AND ASK JESUS TO COME IN AND BE YOUR LORD—LET HIM PUT HIS POSITIVE LIFE WITHIN YOU. LET JESUS COME INTO YOUR HEART.

As an individual receives Jesus Christ as his Lord and personal Savior and lives in daily fellowship with Him, he begins to learn how to put into practice the greatest sermon that was ever preached. The greatest sermon that was ever preached was preached by the Lord Jesus Christ and is known as the Sermon on the Mount (Matthew 5–7). The major portion of this life-centered sermon has to do with human relationships.

Jesus teaches such revolutionary practices as: If anyone strikes on the right cheek, turn to him with the other also; to love, forgive, and bless those who hate you and curse you; to go the second mile with those who force you to go the first mile, and "Pray for those who persecute you!" How contrary all this is to our human nature that wants to hit back harder than we have been hit. Why should we let a negative action by another person dictate how we are going to think, feel, or act.

WITH CHRIST'S HELP, STAND UP AND BECOME A POSITIVE REACTIONARY.
JESUS SAID IT: "OVERCOME EVIL BY DOING GOOD." (See Romans 12:21.)

A Christian's greatest opportunity to witness through the power of Jesus Christ within him is when he is being abused by his fellowman. In the midst of being the victim of the cruelest of personal abuse, when Jesus hung on the cross being crucified, He said, "Father, forgive them; for they know not what they do" (Luke 23:34 KJV). Forgive and do something positive, and no matter what happens, you, too, like Jesus, will be a winner.

4. *Refuse to Surrender the Leadership of Your Life to Negative Circumstances*

A fact of life is that negative things do happen. The car breaks down. Illness comes. Economic conditions change. All these reverses and more are part of our journey here on earth.

But, with Christ's help, you and I do not have to be the victims of circumstances, but we can be the victors over any and all circumstances that come. Speaking of the ups and downs of the economic cycle, a large number of our most profitable businesses in America got their start during the so-called bad times. Why? Because the founders of those businesses refused to surrender the leadership of their lives to bad times. Their belief became stronger; they were more creative; they tried harder; and they refused to give up.

During one of the down cycles economically, there was a man who convinced himself because of bad times, it was impossible for him to succeed in his business.

Caught in the web of negative thinking, he went into a certain shopping center. Fortunately he was still alive enough mentally to observe two different butchers operating out of that same shopping center. One was so busy that people were standing three and four deep to be waited on. The other butcher hardly had any customers at all.

The young man seeking a solution to what he observed decided to investigate. He went into the thriving store, where he waited his turn in line. When it came his turn, the store owner in a polite and courteous manner said, "How do you do? I'm sorry that you had to wait; how can I help you today?" He was positive and congenial and went out of his way to help every customer.

A little later the same day, the young man visited the butcher shop that was failing. Here he found a butcher who growled, "What is it you want?" Instead of giving the young man what he requested, the butcher tried to force another cut upon the unwilling customer. This butcher was negative about everything, and consequently he was reaping negative returns.

Think positive thoughts and you're going to get positive results. But if you think negative thoughts, like the failing butcher, you're going to get negative results. The choice is yours! The Bible gives it to us straight when it says "And as a man thinketh in his heart, so is he" (*see* Proverbs 23:7).

THE WAY TO GET ON TOP OF NEGATIVE CIRCUMSTANCES IS TO CHOOSE TO THINK POSITIVE THOUGHTS. THE CHOICE IS YOURS!

5. Rise up From the Pits and With Positive Thinking Turn Your Minuses Into Pluses

What do you do when life hands you a lemon? With the power of Jesus, you make lemonade. There are scores of people who need a mental resurrection. They are locked into a negative-thinking cycle that is depressing the life right out of them. If, right now, you find that everything looks gloomy, and you find yourself mentally defeated, then you, too, are caught in a negative cycle and you need a new perspective.

The story is told about two boys who were walking down a country road, when they came to a small freight-loading platform on which were two milk cans—to be loaded for delivery in a nearby city.

The boys looked around, and seeing no one, lifted off the cover of can number one and dropped in a big bullfrog. Then they lifted off the cover of can number two and dropped in another bullfrog. The boys continued down the country road, and later the cans were picked up and loaded for city delivery.

During the journey, the bullfrog in can number one said: "This is terrible! I can't lift off the cover of the can because it's too heavy. I have never had a milk bath before, and I can't reach to the bottom of the can to get enough pressure to lift off the cover, so what's the use," and he gave up trying and quit!

When the cover on can number one was taken off, there was a big, dead bullfrog.

The same conditions existed in can number 2, and the frog said to himself: "Well, I can't lift off the cover, because it's too tight and too heavy. I haven't got a brace and bit to drill a hole to save myself, but by the great Father Neptune, there is one thing I learned to do in liquids, and that is to swim." So he swam, and swam, and swam, and churned a lump of butter and sat on it. And when the cover was lifted off, out he jumped, hale and hearty, with the biggest frog broad jump ever recorded in frog history.

*THE WINNER NEVER QUITS—AND THE QUITTER
NEVER WINS!*

WILLIAM E. HOLLER

Jesus is alive—and in the power of the risen Christ you, too, can:

Turn your minuses to pluses
Turn your defeats into victories
Turn your setbacks into advances
Turn bad circumstances into personal growth
Turn failures into successes

6. Dare to Live With Positive Expectation

This past winter, in the midst of a rather prolonged ice storm (of which my wife, Margi, and I were both getting tired), I laughingly said to Margi, "Did you know that spring is coming?" She said, "Doesn't look like spring to me." But I persisted, "That's right! Spring is coming, and before you know it, the flowers will be in full bloom." Somehow just visualizing spring coming made us feel better. One thing about it, when the sun breaks through in the spring-time, we soon forget about all of the struggles of the cold winter. It takes a lot of personal self-discipline to keep looking beyond the hardship to see the positive outcome. The astounding thing is that positive results come to those who stubbornly fix their minds on positive expectation.

The point is, what you anticipate is what you get. Anticipate a great outcome, and you'll get it. Expecting the best acts like a magic magnet, drawing the best to you.

*DISCIPLINE YOURSELF TO KEEP POSITIVE IN A
NEGATIVE WORLD AND YOU WILL NOT ONLY GET
THE BEST, BUT WITH CHRIST'S HELP,
YOU WILL BE
THE BEST YOU CAN BE.
WHAT CAN BE GREATER
THAN TO BE THE BEST YOU CAN BE FOR JESUS?*

DARE TO DISCIPLINE YOURSELF
(No one will ever do it for you!)
God bless you.

ADDITIONAL BOOKS
by the author

Rebuild Your Life
    1975 by Tyndale House Publishers
You Can Win With Love
    1976 by Harvest House Publishers
How to Feel Like a Somebody Again
    1978 by Harvest House Publishers
Expect a Miracle
    1982 by Tyndale House Publishers